# LIVING WITH HIV/AIDS

## THE BLACK PERSON'S GUIDE TO SURVIVAL

Eric Goosby, M. D.

D0126531

Hilton Publishing Company
Roscoe, IL

## Acknowledgments

*Special thanks to Adrianne Appell, whose skill and enterprise were indispensable to the launching of this project.*

Published by Hilton Publishing Company, Inc.
PO Box 737, Roscoe, IL 61073
815-885-1070

www.hiltonpub.com

ISBN: 0-9716067-0-6

# CONTENTS

Contents

# A MESSAGE FROM
# DR. DAVID SATCHER

*Our prevention messages must promote responsible sexual behavior. Quality health care must also be available for those living with HIV/AIDS.*

*To make this happen, we must all take on a role. This includes our families, our friends, our schools, our churches, and our community. In particular, our attitudes—about those most at-risk for HIV and those living with HIV—must be free of negative perceptions and stigma. Because fear of discrimination creates barriers, many individuals may not get tested and learn their status out of fear of being rejected. Persons living with HIV may delay seeking care and may not reach out for the support they need to battle this disease.*

*Finally, I cannot stress enough the disproportionate impact HIV/AIDS is having on minority men, women and children. HIV hits people of color harder than any other segment of the U.S. population. Tackling this national health crisis is most effective at community and individual levels. We must pledge to continue to work together to Educate, Motivate, and Mobilize communities and the public and private sectors in the fight against HIV/AIDS.*

Dr. David Satcher
Former Surgeon General
April 1998

# CHAPTER 1

# PREVENTING THE SPREAD
## What You Must Know

This is the story of a neighborhood and an HIV virus.

Frank has lived in the neighborhood his whole life. Frank shoots heroin. He shares needles. He knows he shouldn't do this, but he is still trying to pretend that he isn't really a drug addict and doesn't need to have his *own* clean needles. One of the people he shares with becomes infected with HIV. Frank shares a needle with this person, as he's shared needles many times in the past, but this time he gets infected.

Frank is infected with HIV but doesn't realize it. He also doesn't realize he can infect others. Frank loves Diane, his live-in girlfriend. They have a child, Charlene.

Diane and Frank don't talk about him being an addict. Diane knows that he uses drugs, but it only comes up as a money issue. Frank is careful not to put his habit in her face. He still thinks of himself as somebody who shoots up only "once in a while." Frank is a good partner, responsive to the needs of Diane and Charlene.

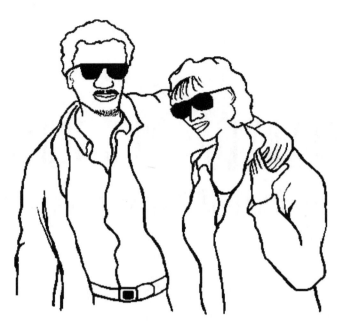

He goes to work every day. Diane doesn't want Frank to think she doesn't trust him. Frank and Diane don't use condoms. Early in their relationship, Diane gets infected.

One night, Frank gets busted. He gets sent to jail. After a month there, he has anal sex with Spence. They don't use a condom. Spence gets infected with HIV. Three months later, Spence gets tested in jail and finds out.

Spence gets out a month later and goes home to his wife, Lisa. They don't use condoms. Spence doesn't feel sick, so he pushes the HIV diagnosis out of his mind until he honestly believes there was a mistake with the HIV test in prison; he doesn't mention it to Lisa. He infects Lisa. Three months later, Lisa is pregnant. Spence is proud and excited to be the father. It's Lisa's first baby. She is so in love. Lisa goes in for routine prenatal blood work. She gets the results back: she is positive for the AIDS virus, HIV. The provider explains to Lisa that she can prevent giving HIV to the baby if she takes a drug called AZT during the pregnancy and during the delivery, and gives it to the baby at birth. But Lisa is so upset by the news that she doesn't keep her follow-up prenatal appointments and is not started on AZT. At the baby's delivery the medical team gives AZT to the baby (whom Lisa and Spence name Louis), but the baby is born with HIV.

Six years later, Diane develops a cough that comes and goes, and feels tired all the time. She has skin rashes on her face and is losing weight. Maybe it's cancer, she thinks. She goes to the clinic. They do blood work. A week later the nurse calls: Diane is sick with HIV; she has AIDS, which is the late stage of HIV. The clinic starts her on drugs for her AIDS, but within two weeks she develops a chronic cough and is short of breath when she walks across the room. She goes to the clinic, where they find she has a kind of pneumonia known as PCP. Diane is admitted to the hospital. While there, she walks through the pediatric ward. She sees a skinny boy playing with blocks. It is Louis, in the hospital for a bad infection.

Diane goes home. She feels like her life is ruined, over. Diane is ashamed and blames herself. She loses hope and doesn't return to the clinic for medication to fight HIV and make her better. One year later, Diane's new boyfriend, Ron, buries her. Ron doesn't think to get tested for HIV. He does-n't feel sick at all.

Six months later, Ron starts dating Cheryl. He infects her with HIV. They have a fight one weekend and Cheryl sleeps with her old boyfriend, Darryl. They don't use condoms. Ron develops a bad cough that won't go away. He drinks cough syrup. He doesn't get tested for HIV. Cheryl finds out she is pregnant. She has prenatal blood work. The results: she has advanced HIV.

This chapter is for everyone — people with HIV, people who love someone with HIV, and people who don't have HIV and want to keep from getting it. It is for people who want the epidemic of HIV in the African American community to stop, and know that the only way to stop it is by learning about it and sharing that knowledge.

## WHY GET TESTED

Every adult should be tested for HIV because you don't really know if you've been exposed to HIV. When you have unprotected sex with someone, you expose yourself not just to that one person, but to everyone that person has had sex with in the past, just as they are exposing themselves to you and your sexual contacts. You may think you know whom you are sleeping with because you trust that person, just as Diane and Lisa trusted their partners. But sometimes trust has nothing to do with it. The truth is that sometimes even your partner may not know if he or she has HIV. Your partner could have been exposed to HIV ten years ago and have no symptoms he or she recognizes as HIV-related.

You should definitely get tested if you have had unprotected sex or have used "needle" (intravenous/IV) drugs in the past or have slept with someone who has used intravenous drugs. You should get tested if you have been in prison and had a sexual encounter or if you have slept with or shared needles with someone who was in prison.

# Facts You Need to Know

According to the most recent National Institutes of Health fact sheet, between 850,000 to 950,000 people in the United States are living with HIV infection. About a quarter of these don't know they're infected. Of the 40,000 new infections that occur each year, 70% are among men, 30% among women. Half of all new cases are people under twenty-five.

Sixty percent of the new infections in men come through homosexual sex, 25% through injection drug use, and 15% through heterosexual sex. Some 50% of the newly infected men are Black, 30% White, and 20% Hispanic, plus a small percentage of other racial/ethnic groups.

The rate of adolescent/adult AIDS cases reported in the United States in 2001 (per 100,000 population) was 76.3 among Blacks, 28.0 among Hispanics, 11.7 among American Indians/Alaska Natives, 7.9 among Whites, and 4.8 among Asians/Pacific Islanders.

The number of new cases among adolescents/adults and the number of new pediatric Aids cases (cases among children under age thirteen) have fallen, but rates among women have increased from 7% to 25% in the years between 1985 and 2001.

Aids is now the fifth leading cause of death in the United States among people twenty-five to forty-four, but among Black men in this age group it is the leading cause of death.

The good news is that the estimated annual number of AIDS-related deaths in the United States fell approximately 70% from 1995 to 2001, from 51,670 deaths in 1995 to 15,603 deaths in 2001. The bad news is that 52% of these deaths were among Blacks.

*You should definitely get tested if you have had unprotected sex or have used "needle" (intravenous/IV) drugs in the past or have slept with someone who has used intravenous drugs. You should get tested if you have been in prison and had a sexual encounter or if you have slept with or shared needles with someone who was in prison.*

Free, anonymous testing is offered in all big cities and most rural areas. Nobody but you will know your results. You can even get tested anonymously by a mail-order kit. (For information on testing, see the Resources section at the end of the book.)

Many tests are available for identifying HIV. Some tests require oral fluid, saliva, urine, finger-stick (blood), or the more common venipuncture. All these tests are looking for HIV antibodies in your blood, urine or oral fluid. Results are generally returned within three weeks.

Understand that most people do not realize they have HIV symptoms. They don't recognize the symptoms of early HIV and feel "symptom free" for as many as fourteen years. Then, they slowly start to get sick. They may get tested at that time. Meanwhile, each person they slept with in the previous decade is at risk of having caught HIV. If you suspect you, or someone you know, may have been exposed to HIV even if they have no symptoms, get tested.

The take-home message is that you don't know your HIV status until you check it. You need to know your status so you can benefit from medical care and take precautions not to infect others. The medical care works, it works in African

# Symptoms That May Mean You Have HIV

Common *Early* Signs Include:

- Feeling tired all the time, even when you get enough sleep
- Painless swelling of your lymph nodes, under your arms, neck, groin
- Frequent skin infections (rashes) on your face, including inside your mouth
- Recurrent colds and herpes outbreaks
- Chronic, long-lasting diarrhea (for weeks)
- Unexplained weight loss
- Recurrent vaginal yeast infections

*Late* Signs of HIV include:

- A dry cough with progressive shortness of breath that lasts for days
- Dark purple swellings on your skin, in your mouth called Kaposi's sarcoma
- Persistent fever with a worsening headache and/or mild confusion
- Inability to use an arm or leg, like a stroke

*Most people do not realize they have HIV symptoms. They don't recognize the symptoms of early HIV and feel "symptom free" for as many as ten years. Then, they slowly start to get sick.*

Americans, it will work in you. It will decrease or eliminate your symptoms; it will usually prolong your life and allow you to look to the future with hope and anticipation once again.

## HOW THE VIRUS IS PASSED

HIV is passed from one person to the next when the blood or bodily fluids of an infected person enters the body of another person. This can happen during vaginal or anal sex, when sharing needles with someone else, or from a transfusion of blood that is contaminated with the virus. The virus enters the body through a puncture, cut, sore or microscopic tear in body tissues, as happens in sex. You may have caught the virus in one of these ways and not know that you are at increased risk for infection.

HIV is hard to get. Casual contact or kissing do not spread the HIV virus. The virus requires contact with body fluids. And the contact has to be through mingling of body fluids. The virus has to get into your body to infect you, through a mucus membrane, cut, infected needle or through contaminated blood products. The virus cannot infect when it is outside the body and exposed to air. You can't get HIV from touching someone who has HIV, from wearing his or her clothes, or from touching a doorknob.

Once you have HIV, you have it. Your symptoms, if untreated, will eventually weaken your immune system, because the HIV is still there. It never goes away.

Myths about HIV abound. One is that you can't get HIV if someone doesn't have any symptoms and looks perfectly healthy. But as I've shown you already, any person who is infected is contagious. This includes people who take the right medications and have the right response to the medications. Though HIV can't be detected in them, they can still infect others.

Another myth is that HIV/AIDS treatment doesn't work in African Americans. This just isn't true. What *is* true is that African Americans are not getting these drugs when they need them. Too often African Americans wait until very late stage disease to begin therapy. These HIV/AIDS drugs work in the African American patient and work well. In my experience with hundreds of African American patients, the drugs are well tolerated, HIV-related symptoms stop, and people who take the medications do well with them and often are able to return to a normal lifestyle, including work.

## HOW HIV IS PASSED SEXUALLY

Let's back up and talk specifically about how HIV can infect you. You get HIV by not wearing a condom when you are having sex. And, if you have HIV now, the only way you can prevent someone else from getting your HIV is if you wear a latex condom when you do have sex. It doesn't matter whether you are straight, gay, male, female, or transgender: the only way to keep others from getting your virus is for you to stop your intimate bodily fluids—semen, blood and vaginal fluid—from getting inside another person. It's that simple. The latex condom does the job.

The phrase, "what goes around, comes around," fits with HIV. Maybe you have HIV and you have unprotected sex with someone, perhaps a stranger. It doesn't seem to matter because you don't know that person and don't care about him or her. But once that person is infected, you never know whom he or she will give the virus to. It could be someone you care about now or will care about in the future.

## HIV TESTING

### When to Get Tested

There are different tests to identify the presence of HIV in a person. Some of the newer tests (viral load, PCR testing, P-24 antigen) show the presence of the virus itself within a few days after infection. Others (EIA, Western Blot, IFA) show the presence of an antibody to HIV, made by the body in response to the presence of the virus. Tests that identify the virus itself are not always available to people who come to a health clinic for HIV testing.

The tests used most commonly to identify HIV-positive people have what is called a "window period." A window period is the period when a person can be infected with HIV but does not test positive because the immune system hasn't

---

*The "window period" is why people are often counseled to wait six weeks until getting tested. If you take the test earlier, it could come out negative, even though you may have HIV and you can infect other people if you have unprotected sex with them.*

---

had enough time to develop an antibody to HIV. The tests used by health departments (EIA and Western Blot) identify the antibody to the most common type of HIV in the United States, called HIV-1. There is another strain of the virus called HIV-2 that is seen in infected people from West Africa.

The "window period" is why people are often counseled to wait six weeks until getting tested. If you take the test earlier, it could come out negative, even though you may have HIV and you can infect other people if you have unprotected sex with them. It would be possible during this window period to get tested using a viral load or P-24 antigen test for HIV-1, which would detect the virus early in the infection before antibody production, but you would have to make special arrangements with your provider.

## Testing Following Unknown Exposure

If you think that you *may* have been exposed to HIV/AIDS, go to a counseling and testing site. Here you will have a private and confidential discussion with an informed professional, who will listen to your concerns and advise you on the best course of action. You will also be offered antibody testing with an EIA screening test. If the results are positive, that will be confirmed with another EIA test; and if that is positive, still a third test called a Western Blot (or in some labs an immuno-fluoresence assay/ IFA) will be done, to make sure it *is* positive. If the Western blot is negative, you will be asked to return in about one month for re-testing. You will also be encouraged to get tested for other sexually transmitted diseases, and you may be referred to a medical clinic.

## Testing Following Known Exposure

How about situations where you know you were exposed recently to a person who is HIV-positive? In such cases, even though your test comes back negative, play it safe and assume you are positive until you have another test (about eight weeks later) that comes back negative. (For more on the primary stage of HIV, see "Post-Exposure Prophylaxis/Pre-Exposure Prophylaxis," on page 28.)

Practice safe sex in the meantime. Use condoms or don't have intercourse, and if you are using IV drugs, don't share needles.

The only time it is safe not to wear a condom is under all three of these conditions:

- You and the other person are not having sex with anyone else
- Neither you nor the other person uses injection drugs
- Both you and the other person have tested negative for HIV (two negative HIV tests for both partners, three months apart)

Remember, eight weeks or a little longer after you have had unprotected sex or shared needles with anyone else, get tested. You'll be giving yourself a chance, and you'll also be giving a chance to others. You will be taking responsibility for yourself and for those you might infect. You'll be part of the solution instead of part of the problem.

If you are HIV-positive and have unprotected sex or share needles, you can be re-infected, by catching a different population of virus. This new population of virus will pose new challenges to your immune system.

In addition, if you are in treatment and already taking anti-retrovirals (ARVs), the new population of HIV may be resistant to the medications you are taking and may not be stopped. This can make you get sicker faster and may make your HIV more complicated to treat.

## OTHER WAYS PEOPLE GET INFECTED

Doctors, nurses, and other hospital workers can, and have, become infected by accidentally sticking themselves with needles or by getting splashes of infected blood into the unprotected eye from patients who were infected with HIV. The stick with an infected needle is more likely to cause infection if the stick is into muscle and draws blood, and if the person by whom the needle was infected had high levels of circulating virus in their blood at that time.

Another way to get infected with HIV is by getting a blood transfusion or receiving a donated body part (e.g. kidney, heart, lung, cornea, tendon) that has not been tested for HIV and that has been infected by the HIV virus. If you are HIV-positive you cannot give blood. The United States Government has required testing of all donated blood since 1984, and has used the P-24Ag test for HIV-1 since the late 1990's. This test identifies people who have been HIV-positive for less than seven days. Thanks to this test, the U.S. blood supply is essentially free of HIV. In other countries, especially countries in sub-Saharan Africa, India, China, and Southeast Asia, transmission of HIV from a blood transfusion is still possible.

Pregnant women can transmit the HIV virus to the growing babies in their wombs, especially if the women are not receiving treatment for HIV. They can also pass the virus to their infants during nursing, by passing the virus through small cuts on their nipples or through their breast milk.

Women commonly don't find out they are infected with HIV until they are pregnant and get an HIV test. If you are pregnant and HIV-positive, you can dramatically improve the chances of having a healthy baby by taking medicines during the pregnancy. The medicines greatly reduce the chance of giving the virus to the baby—from 28% in an untreated HIV-positive mother to less than 5%. Even if you find out just before delivery that you have HIV, you can still take medicines that will offer some protection to your baby. Remember that 65% of the reported cases of AIDS in children are in African American children! This tragedy can be almost completely avoided. (For more on HIV and pregnancy, see chapter 9.)

Finally, it is important for the pregnant HIV-positive mother to get medical attention so she can also take care of herself. Getting a knowledgeable HIV provider, who can help you think through your needs and those of the baby, is critical. With proper

---

*If you are pregnant and HIV-positive, you can dramatically improve the chances of having a healthy baby by taking medicines during the pregnancy. The medicines greatly reduce the chance of giving the virus to the baby—from 28% in an untreated HIV-positive mother to less than 5%.*

---

treatment, progression of HIV in the mother will be slower, and there will be less risk of the mother infecting her baby.

## HIV AND THE PRISONS:
## A REVOLVING DOOR IN THE BLACK COMMUNITY

There are many reasons that HIV has hit Black American communities hard and destroyed entire families, many of them young, just starting out. One of the major reasons is that our young Black men are being put into prisons at an alarming rate. According to Bureau of Justice statistics, Blacks are two times more likely than Hispanics to be in jail, and five times more likely than Whites.

The phenomena of entering prison, getting infected with HIV, and returning to the community is the revolving door of HIV, and one reason for the high rate of HIV in the Black community. But a related reason is that we won't admit that risky behaviors occur in our community. There is a strong stigma against drug abuse, promiscuity, gay sex and a transgender lifestyle in African-American communities. Because of embarrassment and shame associated with these behaviors and lifestyles, people don't want to talk about them, never mind talk about being involved in them.

The shame is often more the fear of shame then the actual shame itself. In actuality, these behaviors are common and tolerated in the wider community, but are almost entirely unspoken of in our community. This silence often prevents individuals from admitting to themselves they are practicing behaviors that could result in getting HIV. This silence is killing our community.

This denial and shame is part of the reason that many men contract HIV in prison. Nobody wants to talk about this but it is true: men locked up with other men have sex together. This is very, very common. Most of these men do not consider themselves gay. But gay or not, when these men don't use condoms, HIV and other diseases spread.

In addition, many people enter prison addicted to IV drugs. Without available drug treatment in prison, they continue to use IV drugs while incarcerated. Needles are often shared in prison settings because it's hard to get clean needles.

Tragically, prison authorities don't like to admit that there is sex and continued drug use occurring in prisons. Because of this silence, prison populations continue to be a major motor for the spread of HIV. Because of their silence, many young Black men, newly infected with HIV, return from prison to their communities. More often then not, released prisoners are

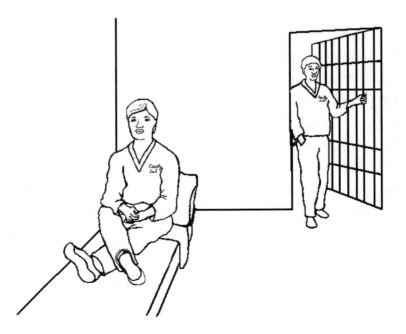

in a state of denial, and do not perceive themselves as having participated in anything that put them at risk for contracting or spreading HIV.

Young men go into prison healthy and come out with HIV. They bring it back to their wives and girlfriends, and to friends they do drugs with. Some of these men were tested in prison and know they have HIV, but they don't tell anyone because they are ashamed of how they got it. They convince themselves that the test result is a mistake.

Others never think about their behavior in prison once they get out. They forget how they took chances and could be infected with HIV. They never get tested, although they participated in very risky behavior. It's as if they think everything that went on is *still* locked up in the prison.

The revolving door between prison and home continues to break dreams and shatter lives in the Black community. People think that what happened in prison won't matter when they get out. But it does. The proof is in the high number of women who get HIV from their men who have been in prison.

HIV can be stopped when people in prison take the same precautions as people out of prison—by using latex condoms and clean needles. Wives and girlfriends should and must insist that their men wear condoms after they get out, no questions asked. Men who have been in prison should get tested immediately after they are freed and again three months later. Until they have two negative HIV tests in a row, and no other exposure to HIV, they should practice safe sex and not share needles. In that way they protect themselves and their loved ones, and help keep HIV from moving through their families and the community.

## THE NEED FOR FRANK TALK

If prison is one of the big causes of the HIV problem, another is our own unwillingness to talk openly about certain sexual issues. Entire families go through life knowing that a son or a brother is gay or transgender, but nobody talks about it openly. The person who is gay or transgender is often afraid of bringing shame on the family, and his or her behavior is driven out of sight.

As long as our community has the misguided belief that it is easier if everyone pretends that the person is not gay or transgender, the risk to the whole community continues. In an atmosphere of community secrecy, the drug user, the gay or transgender person is more likely to stay hidden to society. This means he or she is more likely to catch HIV. He or she is more likely not to seek medical care, where he or she could access drug treatment, and HIV/STD (sexually transmitted diseases) testing, treatment and prevention services. Too often people continue with behaviors that may transmit the virus to others.

Let's be honest, loving someone is often about being willing to have those uncomfortable conversations that are motivated out of concern for the person. The most effective conversations about HIV/AIDS focus on the health/medical issues and *not* about approving or condemning the behavior that may have led to infection. Whether that behavior is intravenous drug use, homosexuality, or a transgender lifestyle, the conversation should, and must, focus on the issue as a disease and on the importance of getting into regular medical care.

What makes this situation tragic is that most families rally around their sons and daughters once they learn their loved one has HIV. They want to help. But people with the disease often conceal it because they fear questions about how they got it, questions that may point to using drugs, or being gay or transgender. They are afraid of the embarrassment to themselves and, even more strongly, to their families.

As mentioned, people in this situation are also less likely to get treatment for HIV because they are afraid that someone will see them. If a man has a girlfriend or wife, he may be afraid to change his behavior in any way—such as using condoms when in the past he has not—that would show that he has HIV. So, while he works out his denial that he has HIV, or the shame he feels or thinks his family will feel if he reveals his behavior(s), he does not take the precautions needed to stop the spread of HIV.

The virus does not discriminate between babies, mothers, teens and fathers; it infects them all. Sometimes men caught up in this net of secrecy don't ask for help until they are in the late stage of disease and can no longer hide it. I have seen families who wait so long that they have to carry their sons to the emergency room for the son's first visit for HIV treatment. Unfortunately, it is long after he had signs of HIV, long after he had unprotected sex, long after he shared needles. Unfortunate, yes, but keep in mind that even at this stage, it is not too late to benefit from medical care.

If you have HIV, be honest about it. Yes this is tough and takes time for everyone, but keep working on it. You have to accept that you are positive before you can take full responsibility for yourself. In rare cases it may even be the correct decision not to reveal yourself to family or friends. But talk to someone. If you don't want to tell people you may be infected, give their names to your provider, and the provider can tell them.

Be honest enough with yourself not to infect anyone else and to protect yourself from picking up more HIV. Make sure to have condoms on hand for any occasion where you might have sex. If you shoot drugs, don't shoot with dirty needles, don't share needles. The most important thing is to get medical care for HIV, for your sake. HIV is a lifelong illness and requires that you get medical care—from a knowledgeable provider for life.

*You have to accept that you are positive before you can take full responsibility for yourself.*

# CHAPTER 2

# WHAT IS HIV?
# WHAT IS AIDS?

*Medical literacy is the missing link in quality health care.*
—Neil Shulman ("Doc Hollywood"), M. D.

AIDS, or Acquired Immune Deficiency Syndrome, is caused by a virus. Understanding the virus will give you a better idea of what to expect from the disease. But even more importantly, by learning about the virus, you will feel more comfortable speaking with your provider about your illness, test results and treatment. Once you can begin to speak the language of HIV, you'll be in a better position to ask questions and to choose options among treatments. Understanding HIV will open up many other resources to you, such as magazines, Internet web sites and books. In short, you will be able to better ensure that you get the best treatment available.

Knowledge is power. People with HIV have shown this to be true over and over again. In the 1980s, groups of people with HIV educated themselves about their disease and used that information to demand more research, better treatment and more money to care for people with HIV. This group of highly informed HIV-positive patients, partners and friends demanded that the medical systems delivering care be informed and guided by their input. It changed the way medicine was, and is, practiced, not only for HIV but most chronic progressive diseases.

*By learning about the virus, you will feel more comfortable speaking with your provider about your illness, test results and treatment.*

The African American community does not fully benefit from what the medical system can offer. African Americans with HIV and most other medical illnesses have not taken advantage of preventive medical care because we so often are not being followed by a doctor, nurse provider or other health professional. The variables that make it harder for some people to get medical help than others are well known. Certainly, costs always serve as a barrier. But it is not just issues of access to health care and cost. It is much more complicated. It has to do with how we look at health care, and how we feel about our right to access it as a community.

Many times our people have failed to take advantage of available health care. Too many times our elderly have not acted, even when they were suffering from severe symptoms, such as shortness of breath, chest pain, and difficulty urinating or unexplained weight loss. They simply did not seek out the health care that was readily available to them. With HIV, I have seen people of all ages ignore severe symptoms for months to years, until they had to enter health care through the emergency room with a life-threatening infection.

It is important to ask ourselves why this is the case. It is something only we can address for ourselves. We are the only ones who can change the expectation in our community that it is acceptable to endure a symptom, that it is acceptable not to seek medical help. We have to start challenging excuses such as, "I can't afford it," "hospitals are a place to go to die," "medicines don't work on Black people," or "they will experiment on me if I go to the hospital."

If equal quality in health care is a political problem, it is also a problem for each community and individual to address, and the first step is getting the necessary knowledge. So let's begin by learning something about what happens when the HIV virus enters your body.


## THE NATURAL HISTORY OF HIV

The HIV virus is ruthlessly efficient at invading and taking over a human body. Like other viruses, HIV uses the cells of your body to reproduce itself. But in the case of HIV, the virus takes over the very cells your body uses to fight infections like HIV—the cells of the immune system. Your immune system is a remarkable defensive force that not only fights off minor diseases like colds but also helps you resist major ones like tuberculosis and cancer. If the immune system is undermined, you become susceptible to all kinds of disease.

HIV, the virus that causes AIDS, is a type of virus that contains genetic material composed of ribonucleic acid (RNA). Genes provide a blueprint for your life, determining everything from the color of your hair or skin to your body's ability to fight off disease. It is unusual for a virus to use RNA as genetic material to produce and duplicate cells—most use DNA (deoxyribonucleic acid). The use of RNA as genetic material requires an extra step for the successful takeover of the host cell: the RNA must be changed into DNA. Such a virus is called a *retrovirus*, because, in a way, it's backward: it requires RNA to change to DNA instead of the usual DNA to RNA.

HIV is simply composed of its outer shell and projections, or spikes, that attach to the outside surface of the host cell (the cell the virus is infecting). The outside shell of the HIV virus looks like a soccer ball covered with many small spikes. The virus searches for specific receptors, or landing sites, on the surface of the host cell. The HIV virus likes to attach itself specifically to a site called CD4. There are many CD4 landing sites on each host cell. After attaching onto one of the immune cells on the CD4 receptor site, the virus injects its genetic material into the cell. Once the HIV virus's RNA is in the cytoplasm of the cell (the material that surrounds the nucleus or center), it is transformed into DNA by the action of an enzyme called Reverse Transcriptase.

The newly formed DNA moves to the nucleus, or core, of the host cell. The nucleus is full of genetic material. The viral DNA mixes with the host cell DNA by the action of an enzyme called "integrase." This allows new virus particles to be made while using the host cell's own machinery.

This infection process results in the production of thousands of unassembled virus particles. When these virus particles are assembled, they form a whole new HIV called a "virion," through the action of another enzyme called "protease." Once assembled, the virions burst the cell wall of the host cell and move to identify adjacent cells containing CD4 receptor sites. This process repeats over and over. That's how the virus multiplies and eventually thrives. It uses your cells.

You can understand many of the symptoms caused by HIV by understanding which cells have CD4 receptors on their surfaces, marking them for attack by the invading virus or virions.

- When cells that insulate the nerves in your hands and feet are infected by HIV, you feel burning, numbness or tingling.
- When the epithelial cells that line your colon are infected with HIV, you get chronic diarrhea.
- When infected epithelial cells are found in your skin, you get recurrent rashes on your face and trunk.
- When the glial cells in the brain (the cells that allow the neurons to work) are infected, you may get accelerated dementia (slowed thinking, recurrent forgetfulness of recent events).

## Your Immune System Response to HIV

What does your immune system do while the HIV virus is setting up shop in cells in your body that contain CD4 receptor sites? Well, your immune system goes into high gear, and releases a variety of white blood cells into your bloodstream to try to kill the invader. The immune system tries to attack the HIV cells directly with white cells specifically designed to identify an invading foreign organism and contain it.

Once the invader is contained, the immune system sends large cells in to eat the debris left over from the fight between your white cells and the HIV virus. Unfortunately, the HIV virus can make hundreds of thousands of virions, all of which are capable of infecting other cells.

The virus's fight with the body's immune system kills and replaces thousands of your immune cells, including the entire population of cells that direct the immune response, (CD4 T lymphocytes) every forty-eight hours. About two weeks after being infected, you may feel sick, as if you had the flu. Most people do not recognize these flu-like symptoms as the first sign of HIV infection. Medically, we do recognize this early stage as Primary HIV syndrome (see page 27). Your body can keep up this intense immune response for about eight to ten years; then its ability to replace the destroyed CD4 T-lymphocytes is compromised. By this time, the total number of CD4-containing T-cells have dwindled down.

Your ability to fight infections is adequate until you reach a level of 200 CD4 cells. When you have fewer than 200 CD4 cells, the frequency of life-threatening infections increases. That's when HIV symptoms become more severe, and, unfortunately, that is when we often see people who have ignored their HIV for years coming into the emergency room with symptoms of their first life-threatening infection.

## Primary HIV Syndrome

The first signs and symptoms you get after being infected with the HIV virus for the first time are known as the Primary HIV Syndrome. This syndrome usually occurs seven to fourteen days after exposure and lasts for twenty-one days. It is important to recognize for two big reasons: you are now infected with the HIV virus and can infect other people; if you get it diagnosed now, it is possible to give you a short course of anti-retroviral (ARV) drugs. Research shows that such treatment, given as long as two years after you were infected, may slow the progression of HIV in your body in the coming years.

It is important for you to know about this Primary HIV Syndrome so you can talk to your health care provider about the potential benefits, and risks, of a short course of antiretro-virals. Most people are given a six-month course, and then stop, but the length of time you need to take medication must be a decision made between you and your provider.

What are the symptoms of Primary HIV syndrome? You may have:

- Fever
- Rash
- Muscle aches and pain
- Swollen lymph nodes (glands)
- Headache
- Sensitivity to light
- Yeast infection called *thrush* (a white patch that doesn't brush off) on the tongue and in the mouth

It is important to know that at this stage of the infection, some people feel very sick and others hardly notice what is happening. The symptoms generally last for fourteen to twenty-one days. After that, the symptoms go away and the virus enters a "latency," or quiet, phase.

But the virus has not gone away. It continues to attack your immune cells. You may have no obvious symptoms, but the HIV is active in your body and your body is still trying to fight the virus. It's a silent battle that can last for ten years or more, and you may or may not know you have the virus. You remain infected, however, and contagious. You must practice safe sex and not share needles so you won't infect others.

If you suspect that you or a friend may have become infected with HIV less than six months ago, you or your friend may also benefit from a shortened course of antiretroviral drugs, just as if you had been diagnosed for a first stage HIV infection. The earlier the HIV is treated, the better. It makes no sense to play Russian roulette with HIV.

## Post-Exposure Prophylaxis/Pre-Exposure Prophylaxis

"Prophylaxis" means prevention of disease. Though the final answer isn't in, studies on health care workers known to have been exposed suggest that HIV infection may be prevented by taking a four-week course of antiretroviral medications after an exposure. Taking ARV as close to the time of exposure as possible may prevent the virus from anchoring in your cells and thus prevent infection and the development of antibodies.

Researchers have begun to look at giving ARVs to people after sexual exposure, such as rape, and to some health care workers before exposure (pre-exposure prophylaxis) as a preventative measure. Further research is needed to clarify when the use of ARVs is indicated.

What *is* clear is that you should talk to your health care provider as soon as possible if you think you have been exposed to someone with HIV.

# CHAPTER 3

# YOUR FIRST VISIT TO THE HEALTH CARE PROVIDER

## STAGING HIV

After you test positive for HIV, your provider will want to run tests to check your overall health, to see how much of the virus is in your body and whether it has caused damage, and also to stop any infections you may already have. This is called "staging" the disease.

Get ready. You may be in for a long visit, involving blood drawing, baseline X rays, urine tests and a pelvic examination. The tests are sometimes done in one long day, sometimes over several visits. But either way, these tests are important and will let your health care provider know just how advanced your infection is and develop a plan that meets all your needs.

Some people feel that all this attention is an intrusion. People will be touching you, probing you and sticking you with needles, all this right after you learned you have a serious disease and feel especially vulnerable. But hang in there, and get it done. You know that your life depends on it.

The reason there are so many tests is simple: HIV is a complicated disease that can involve different areas of your body. This is why it is important to be thorough in evaluating the extent of disease at the outset: it allows you and your provider to decide on the exact treatment(s) you need. Because of the HIV, you may have any of a number of symptoms or illnesses—symptoms you didn't realize were related to HIV, such as a rash or a vaginal infection. If you skip a scheduled chest X ray, for example, and you are harboring a lung disease, the disease can quickly land you in the hospital or worse.

If you need motivation to go through with the tests, draw strength from the knowledge that many others have been through the same process: 37% of the approximately 900,000 people living with HIV in the United States are African American. Among newly infected men in this country, 50% are Black, and among newly infected women, 64% are Black. Only when more of us get tested and follow up on our visits and treatment can we begin to change these statistics.

So you have a lot of reasons to get to the provider, get tested, and get appropriate treatment. By doing so you ensure that:

- The disease in you will progress more slowly
- You won't get as many infections
- The infections you do get will be less severe
- You will prolong your life
- You will help slow the spread of this disease in our community

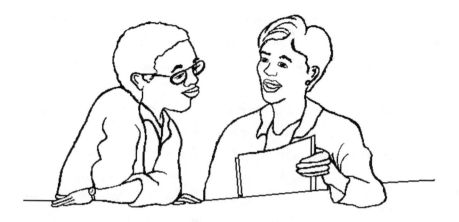

Also, your actions may help someone you care about from getting HIV, or keep an HIV-positive child from catching an infection you are harboring. Maybe you will inspire people you know to go through with HIV testing and treatment. By getting tests yourself, you become part of a movement to hold HIV/AIDS in check and eventually to defeat it altogether. You help your community.

*You may feel more comfortable having a friend or family member with you when you have the tests done.*

You may feel more comfortable having a friend or family member with you when you have the tests done. You may feel overwhelmed by learning you are HIV-positive and you may not be thinking very clearly about anything else. This is normal! So bring a friend with you, perhaps someone who has gone through the experience already and knows exactly what you are going through.

During the visit to your health care provider, your friend can worry about appointments, phone numbers, transportation and paperwork, and you can concentrate on getting to know your provider. If you want to have a friend present, tell the nurse and schedule your tests for a day when your friend can go with you.

Whether you take a friend with you or not, before your appointment, write down any questions or concerns you have, and bring this paper with you. On the day of the tests, you may be so stressed out that you forget the questions you wanted to ask. A list can help you remember to ask the questions that are important to you. It often helps to create a permanent diary of questions, issues and concerns that you can refer to over a series of visits. Purchasing a spiral binder in the grocery store will do the trick.

*Before your appointment, write down any questions or concerns you have, and bring this paper with you.*

At your visit, the provider will probably ask you many personal questions about your lifestyle (including questions about your sex life and whether you need to go through drug or alcohol detox), along with questions about your general health and any symptoms you are having. Depending on your symptoms and the results of your tests, the provider may start you on drugs to help you fight the virus and help you feel better. It is important to be honest, even though it may be embarrassing.

You will encounter a number of health care people during the tests—doctors, nurse practitioners, and physician's assistants. But there will probably be one person other than your primary care provider with whom you will develop an ongoing relationship. This person, called a "case manager," is responsible for coordinating your care between your provider and other consultants. The case manager doesn't take the place of your primary provider, but helps with the logistics of getting your tests and consultations completed and gets back to your provider about the results. The case manager may also play a role in talking to you about the importance of taking your medications, and about behaviors that decrease or eliminate the chance of you spreading the virus to others.

At a clinic, your first meeting will probably be with a nurse. He or she may review with you the tests you are about to get. You probably will have an opportunity to ask him or her many questions about HIV and your health. This is the time to ask about safe sex practices. Don't be embarrassed. The HIV nurse's main job is educating patients about HIV, including safe sex. They have heard it all!

The embarrassing questions will only be asked once. You won't have to answer them again. Your nurses are not interested in your private life. Their job is to help slow the spread of disease in you and also in your community. It's important that we, as a community, understand how the virus moves from one person to another, and it's part of the HIV nurse's job to help us understand that and thus help protect one another from new infection. Remember that the nurse will not reveal to anyone any of the information you tell him or her without your expressed permission. Often patients want or need help telling others they may have been exposed to infection; in this situation a plan is worked out that you control.

*Your nurses are not interested in your private life. Their job is to help slow the spread of disease in you and also in your community.*

Next, the health care provider will begin your exam and begin arranging for your various tests. The good news is that if you are having any problems now—a troublesome skin infection or ear or eye problems, for example—help is on the way. Tell the provider about any problems you are having, even if you don't think they are related to the HIV. With HIV, small problems can build quickly and you want to catch them early.

HIV can be a harsh disease, yes, but you don't need to suffer! Medicines and people are available to help. You just need to ask for them.

To begin, you will be given a general physical exam in which your blood pressure will be checked and heart and lungs listened to. The provider will ask you about any symptoms you are having. He or she will also check for typical signs of HIV involving your skin, fingertips, lungs, mouth and eyes. Women may receive a gynecological exam and, if indicated, a pregnancy test.

The provider will examine your skin and feet for skin cancer, herpes, fungal or bacterial infections or dry, inflamed patches of psoriasis. If you have any of these conditions and are uncomfortable, the provider can give you creams to ease the discomfort or treat the infection.

Your throat will be examined for signs of thrush, a yeast infection that looks like a white patch on your tongue and roof of your mouth. It usually is not painful and is easily treated. Your mouth will be examined for other infections, including oral hairy leukoplakia, and a type of skin cancer common in HIV called Kaposi's sarcoma.

The nurse may draw your blood or direct you to a clinic to have this done. The general health of your blood will be examined to determine:

- How many red and white cells you have
- The amount of fat, cholesterol and triglycerides
- Kidney function and liver function
- Signs of diabetes
- Evidence of past infections such as syphilis; hepatitis A, B, C; toxoplasmosis (see "other blood tests" on page 42); and tuberculosis (PPD and/or X ray)

It is important to identify evidence of past infections as well as current ones, so a treatment plan that addresses all your needs can be presented to you in your next visit.

Two very important tests you will have done many times during the next few years are the following:

- CD4 test
- Viral load

They show how well your body is fighting the HIV infection and help the health care provider determine what stage your disease is in. The provider reviews these tests and your symptoms to decide whether it is the right time to offer you medication for the HIV. With the text results in hand, the provider can help give you a general idea of how long you may have had the HIV infection and how close you may be to developing a diagnosis of AIDS. These tests are important, so let's talk about each of them.

## THE CD4 TEST

The CD4 test shows how strong your immune system is by counting the number of CD4 cells you have. What is a CD4 cells? A CD4 cell is a type of white blood cell, called a "helper T-cell," that fights infections. When HIV invades the body, the virus heads straight for the T-cells and begins to take them over and destroy them. Your body fights back by producing more T-cells. At first your body stays ahead of the virus. As the virus destroys cells, your body makes new ones. But after a while, about eight years later, your body gets tired and can't keep up. The virus keeps destroying cells but your body can't make enough to replace them. This lower number of CD4 cells shows up on a CD4 test.

The helper T-cell is one of many types of white blood cells that fight infection. So, even with a low CD4 cell count, part of your immune system is still functioning. But overall, if you have HIV, your immune system is impaired. The CD4 cells are the alarm ringers—they watch for infections that invade the body, and alert the rest of your immune system when that happens. When you have fewer CD4 cells because of HIV, it is more difficult for your body to know when an infection has entered your body because there are fewer "alarm ringers," so it is also harder for the body to defend itself.

A healthy person without HIV has 600 to 1,500 CD4 cells per microliter of blood. People fighting hard against HIV may show an upper level of 600 CD4 cells about five years after being infected, 520 after eight years, and 440 after nine years. This drop is about 80 CD4 cells each year. Other people may have begun their HIV infection at a starting CD4 count of

1,500. Their decline over the same period of time may show a CD4 count of 1,100. Severe symptoms begin at a CD4 of 200 or less.

Some clinics (especially pediatric clinics) also measure CD4 cells as a percentage of CD4 cells to the total lymphocyte count. In a healthy person, 20 percent to 40 percent of T-cells are CD4 cells. Someone with HIV will have a smaller percentage of CD4 cells to the total lymphocyte count. The CD4 count also may be reported to you as a ratio of CD4 cells to another type of T-helper cell called a CD8+ cell. The results are given as a single figure that tells how many CD4 cells are present for each CD8 cell. A healthy person has a ratio of 0.9 to 1.9. Someone with HIV may have a ratio as small as 0.4.

When your health care provider reviews your CD4 count for the first time, he or she may be able to say how close you are to having complications due to HIV, but it will be only a guess. Nobody knows when your CD4 count will drop to the point where you will have symptoms. It varies from person to person. Some people have a strong CD4 count for years, and then it drops suddenly, often during an intercurrent infection. Stress and other infections can cause your CD4 count to drop. Your CD4 count will probably come back up after the infection is cleared up. This is a normal and expected response to any infection for HIV-infected and non-HIV infected people.

Most people do not know for sure when they were infected with HIV. Taking a CD4 count every three to six months can alert you and your health care provider to a change in your HIV infection before you see or feel any new symptoms.

When you return for future CD4 tests, the clinic will probably recommend that you have blood drawn at about the same time of day each visit. The reason is that CD4 counts go up and down during the day, for healthy people and those with HIV. So, if you can, try to schedule all of your appointments for tests at roughly the same time of day.

*Taking a CD4 count every three to six months can alert you and your provider to a change in your HIV infection before you see or feel any new symptoms.*

## VIRAL LOAD TEST

The second test mentioned, the viral load, is a rough measure of the number of virus particles in a milliliter of your blood. The HIV virus hides out and reproduces in your immune cells and tissue, but it also circulates in your blood. The stronger the HIV virus, the more of it there is in your blood. A person who is not infected with HIV will have no HIV virus particles in his or her blood. Someone with HIV may have a viral load of less than 40 copies per milliliters or more than 500,000 copies per milliliter.

With antiretroviral therapy, people with HIV can lower their viral load to 10,000 or 5,000, or even to a value so low that it can't be detected. At that point, it is called "undetectable." This confuses some people into believing that the virus is gone. But the virus in still in the body, though at so low a level in the blood that the test can't pick it up. Also, as we know, the virus likes to live inside cells. It conceals itself, but it is still there. The cells it hides in include cells in the lymph nodes (glands), liver, spleen, brain and bone marrow.

Researchers have been frustrated because the cells in which it hides give the virus shelter from the antiretroviral drugs that can kill it.

The results of the viral load test, in combination with the CD4 test, and your medical history, are used to determine what stage your HIV infection is in. If you have a high viral load, meaning there is a lot of virus in your blood, but a high CD4 count, it may mean that you are early in the infection cycle (recently infected). The virus is reproducing but, so far, your body has been able to make enough extra CD4 cells to keep up with the number being destroyed.

There are two ways to do a viral load test:

1)  A bDNA test
2)  A PCR test

In the United States, the test results are reported in the same units. Regular PCR has a lower limit of detection of 400 viral copies per milliliter, whereas the newly developed ultra-sensitive assay has a lower limit of detection of 40 copies per milliliter. The other two assays are a branched DNA (bDNA) assay and a nucleic acid sequence amplification assay. For your own treatment, it is important that your provider be aware of the different test types you have used, so accurate comparisons can be made.

Any acute infection, such as flu, or immunization, such as pneumovax, may temporarily change your viral load. It is recommended that you wait three to four weeks after an infection or immunization, before having a viral load test.

|  | Early | Middle | Late |
|---|---|---|---|
| **Viral Load** | high | high | high |
| **CD4** | high | medium | low |

## OTHER BLOOD TESTS

During your first few visits, the health care provider will run a number of other tests, in addition to the CD4 and viral loas tests. Your blood will be tested for evidence of other infections that people who are HIV-positive often get. The reason this is important is that these other diseases progress much more rapidly in someone with HIV. Such infections can include syphilis, hepatitis A, hepatitis B, hepatitis C. If you are an IV drug user, it is highly likely you have hepatitis C. If you do, it requires immediate diagnosis and consideration for treatment, whether or not you begin treatment of your HIV.

Hepatitis A, B, and C are treatable. Hepatitis B and C are serious, chronic diseases that can destroy your liver. A healthy liver is needed in order to live well. Your provider must decide how the presence of a chronic Hepatitis B or C infection will influence the choice of antiretroviral medications as well as the need for specific treatment for the hepatitis B and C. You may not have any symptoms of Hepatitis B or C.

Your blood also will be tested for syphilis and "toxoplasmosis." (Toxoplasmosis may occur in the late stages of HIV.) The health of your kidney and liver will also be checked through blood tests and monitored over time. Since some of the antiretroviral drugs cause the blood lipids (fats) to rise, your cholesterol and triglycerides will be checked to establish a baseline value (this should be done after a twelve-hour fast). In addition, a fasting blood glucose level may be checked to identify early diabetes mellitus.

## TUBERCULOSIS

You also will be given a PPD test (Purified Protein Derivative) for tuberculosis (TB). Tuberculosis is a disease that often runs hand in hand with HIV and can occur at any T-cell count. TB can involve any organ system, but it most often involves the lungs.

The PPD test is simple. The nurse will inject a small amount of PPD into your forearm and within forty-eight to seventy-two hours, if you have been exposed to TB and your CD4 cells are not too low, it will show up as a small but raised bump in the area of the injection. You may be asked to return to the clinic in two or three days so the nurse can check the result of the TB-PPD test. If it is considered positive, you will need a chest X ray to make sure there is no evidence of "active disease."

TB is an organism that gets into your body if you inhale small droplets of mucus that contain TB. Your body will respond to the organism in the lungs by surrounding it with white cells and containing the infection. If your body's response is successful, the initial infection with TB will not lead to active disease. Instead, you will have stopped the infection from progressing to an active case. This means you were infected with TB but stopped the infection early. People who stop the infection often "reactivate" with TB when their immune systems are weakened, such as occurs with old age, cancer or HIV.

If you have a positive PPD and a normal chest X ray, you will need to take a drug called "isoniazide" (INH) with a B-6 vitamin called "pyradoxine." You'll need to take it for a period of at least twelve months; some experts recommend taking it for life. If you have active disease, you will need a combination of drugs for a nine-month period to effectively treat TB. These drugs are complicated and have many potential interactions with HIV medications. Your health care provider will orchestrate how many you take and the dose you need. The important thing to remember is that TB commonly runs with HIV and if TB is identified, it is fully treatable.

*The important thing to remember is that TB commonly runs with HIV and if TB is identified, it is fully treatable.*

## OTHER IMPORTANT TESTS

You may be given an eye exam to make sure you are not suffering eye problems due to an eye disease associated with HIV called cytomegalovirus (CMV). This disease is seen in patients with very low CD4 counts (less than one hundred). The health care provider may put drops in your eyes to dilate, or open, your pupils. This allows him to examine the back of your eye (called the retina). The retina is where the optic nerve enters your eye and is the site where CMV likes to grow.

Because it has a characteristic appearance in the back of the eye, CMV involvement of the retina is often diagnosed by visual examination of the retina in the office. The provider cannot see your entire retina, and so patients with CD4 counts below 1,200 may be referred to an ophthalmologist, an eye specialist. The ophthalmologist has an instrument that can examine all areas of your retina that could be infected with CMV.

You may be given vaccines against the flu, Hepatitis A and Hepatitis B if your blood work shows no evidence of your having had these infections already and your T-cells are not too low. In addition you should receive the routine vaccine for diphtheria and tetanus every ten years. You should also be given a vaccine called pneumovax which will protect you from a common cause of death in AIDS patients, bacterial pneumonia. Vaccines work better in people with higher numbers of T-cells (greater than 500 cells per microliter), but should be offered to people with low numbers of T-cells (even as low as 200 cell per microliter).

You may be asked for a urine sample, to check for sugar, protein or bacteria, to make sure you don't have a bladder or kidney infection and that your kidneys are working well.

## IF YOU ARE FEMALE

If you are female, you will be given a gynecological exam during which a Pap smear will be taken. The Pap smear is a test for the abnormal cervical cells that can develop into cancer of the cervix. In addition, tests can be done to identify human papilloma virus (HPV), which commonly causes cancer of the cervix. In HIV-positive women, the virus is more common and stronger.

You may be checked for infections, including a yeast infection caused by candida albicans, which also is common in HIV-positive women. Checking for pregnancy may also occur at this time. The most common test is the pregnancy urine test, but there are also blood tests that pick up very early pregnancies. A discussion about birth control needs is also important and should take place at this time.

## YOUR TEETH

If you haven't seen a dentist in a while, you may be directed to one, especially if you have painful, bleeding gums. With HIV, you may not have a strong enough immune system to fight minor bacterial infections in your mouth, especially those that cause plaque. It is normal to have bacteria in the mouth and people with healthy immune systems keep these bacteria under control. With HIV, the bacteria can take over and cause painful, bleeding gums and infection that can spread into your jaw and make you feel run down. The dentist also may check your mouth for Kaposi's sarcoma.

## YOUR SOCIAL WORKER OR CASEWORKER

You may be directed to a social worker or caseworker, who can help with concerns or stresses in your life about your living situation or your finances. These stresses can affect your health (see Chapter 13, "Stress and Stress Relief.").

If you are an IV drug user or you abuse alcohol, the social worker may try to find you a spot in a detox program. Addiction doesn't mean you can't be treated for HIV. You can. It does mean you will be encouraged to get clean. If you begin on methadone for heroin addiction, or are on methadone now, this treatment must be coordinated with your HIV treatment, because the methadone can interact with some HIV drugs. (For more about addiction and HIV, turn to Chapter 11.)

The social worker may help with other stresses, including transportation to the health care provider, clothes or daycare for your children while you are seeing your provider. This is your opportunity to identify those things in your life that cause you stress. Take advantage of it! It is the social worker's job to assist you. Life is hard. Accept the help that is offered. Less stress in your life means you will have a higher CD4 count and will be healthier.

Good nutrition and your ability to eat well are critical to staying well. The social worker may check to see if you have access to a kitchen and adequate cooking supplies, if you need assistance from a food pantry, or would like to see a dietitian to help you learn how to make healthy meals for yourself and your family.

The social worker may ask if you are interested in receiving regular counseling with an expert who can help you or your family sort out your feelings about HIV. Don't be offended! If anything in life is stressful, finding out you have HIV is. The counselor can help you sort out your feelings and arrange the other details of your life to accommodate your HIV.

Most patients get the most relief from peer-run support groups—that is, from others who have HIV. These groups help cut through the isolation you may feel. You will find that you are not alone, and that many other people share your concerns and your symptoms. These peers also can be a great source of information about what you can expect from living with HIV and about other resources in your community that are available to you.

## THE TEST RESULTS

If your health care provider does not use the "Rapid HIV Test" you may not get the results of your HIV test for a week or more. When it comes back from the lab, your team—the provider, nurse, case manager and social worker—will sit down and come up with a proposed plan for treating your HIV. When you return for your follow-up appointment with the nurse, she will tell you the test results and what tests or treatment the team thinks is best for you.

It is not uncommon to be very anxious and worried at this time. If you are concerned, you should seek help by calling the health care provider or social worker. They are prepared to help. They are there to help. Before you leave from your first testing visit, make sure you know whom to call after hours if you need to, and get that person's or organization's phone number. Someone will be there to listen to you. If you are connected to a church or know of an AIDS ministry, this is the time to seek counseling and encouragement from a pastor.

It is normal to feel very nervous and scared after you have been told you are HIV-positive. Maybe you were too shaken to ask questions. Hang in there! Questions that you did not ask during your visit will come to mind later. Don't hesitate to call your provider. They expect and welcome it.

Remember that you are not alone. Hundreds of thousands

---

*It is not uncommon to be very anxious and worried. If you are concerned, you should seek help by calling the health care provider or social worker. They are prepared to help. They are there to help.*

of other people have gone through the same tests and challenges, and come through them stronger than before.

At this point your health care team has reviewed your symptoms and looked at the results of all your tests, including the viral load and CD4. In this way they will determine what stage your HIV infection is in and how strong your immune system is.

> *Remember that you are not alone. Hundreds of thousands of other people have gone through the same tests and challenges, and come through them stronger than before.*

If you have no symptoms, a low viral load and strong CD4 results (greater than 350), the provider may tell you that your immune system is strong and that you still have time before you need any therapy. You may be HIV-positive but, since you have no symptoms and require little or no treatment with medications, you may simply be advised to focus on getting your immunizations up to date.

If it appears from your symptoms or test results that the HIV infection is stressing your immune system, your provider may tell you that you would benefit from medications that will prevent opportunistic infections (infections that can result from your weakened immune system). If your immune system is very weak, the provider may tell you that you have AIDS. Don't despair! You can get a better quality of life with treatment and, by paying close attention to your care, can expect to live for many years to come. Good productive years. We now have effective drugs that can slow the progression of the disease. You can take these drugs. Instead of one infection and hospitalization after another, you can live well.

## YOUR PART IN THE PLAN

When the health care provider tells you about the proposed treatment plan, speak up about what you don't understand. If something in the plan sounds like it won't work for you, tell the provider so he or she can make a change. For example, maybe your team believes you should come to the "Tuesday" HIV clinic every three months to have your CD4 checked. Tuesdays, however, you work and can't get off. Ask the nurse if you can come to the Wednesday evening clinic instead.

Or maybe the team will recommend that you start on anti-retroviral therapy immediately. But you are basically feeling O.K. and want to delay for a few months until summer vacation is over and your son is back in grade school. You are afraid that you may have a hard time with the side effects and you don't want to have to juggle the new drugs with work and taking care of your son. Ask the provider if you can delay treatment for a few months. Don't be afraid. Be clear on what is being planned for you, but know that it is *your* plan and needs to address *your* needs, not just the needs of the system caring for you. Make your plan work for you, so you will be able to stick with it and get as healthy as you can.

# CHAPTER 4

# RESPONSIBILITIES

In this book we encourage you to use your HIV diagnosis as an opportunity to take good care of yourself and to get the good medical care that you deserve. This means taking on a new set of responsibilities, like eating well, getting rest and taking any medications your provider has prescribed.

You may feel overwhelmed by it all. You may have children or parents you care for, a job, rent or a mortgage to pay, a spouse, a drug or alcohol habit you are trying to beat. There is a lot on your shoulders! Try to understand that your new life with HIV doesn't mean that your old life is over. It really is a chance to make a new beginning and change those problems in your life that need to be changed. It may be difficult at first, but try to be optimistic about your life.

Believe it or not, these responsibilities may be easier to bear when you are feeling good about yourself and are taking good care of yourself.

We know how easy it can be for you to feel bad about yourself at a time like this, blaming yourself for your illness. Don't go there! It is destructive to your spirit. It is a dead-end road.

> *We know how easy it can be for you to feel bad about yourself at a time like this, blaming yourself for your illness. Don't go there! It is destructive to your spirit.*

When people feel this way, they have little desire to take good care of themselves or to be responsible toward others. Try to use the intensity of your feelings as positive motivation to take care of yourself.

If you don't feel like you deserve good care, you are not going to seek it out. If you feel ashamed of yourself for being HIV-positive—perhaps afraid that people will criticize you for having gay sex, being promiscuous, being transgender, being in a "bad" relationship, using drugs or abusing alcohol—this feeling alone can drive you to behaviors that are destructive to you and others.

You may pretend that you do not care about yourself and others, and continue to have sex without using a condom. You *do* care and you are kidding yourself to believe otherwise. You can deny now that you care but at some point you will have to face your feelings of how much you do care about yourself, your loved ones and your community.

---

*Taking good care of yourself also means doing right by your family, your friends and your community. It means doing your part to end HIV infection among Black Americans.*

---

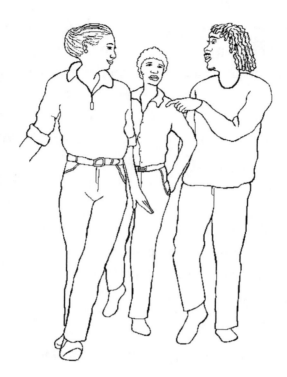

Negative feelings often go along with the tendency to shrug off responsibilities. This is one primary reason why the epidemic of HIV continues to rage through Black communities across our nation. So taking good care of yourself also means doing right by your family, your friends and your community. It means doing your part to end HIV infection among Black Americans.

If you are like most people with HIV and AIDS, you will work through your fears and get into a new rhythm. Everything in your life that you enjoy doing and that gives you energy will still be available to you. Don't believe your life has stopped with a diagnosis of HIV. It is true your life will need to change, but it does not need to stop. Take pleasure in the things that don't have to change—your job, the house you live in, the pleasure of spending time with family and friends.

The key is to find and strengthen the ways you have to feel good about yourself. We're not talking about the *old* quick fixes—eating ice cream sundaes or going out and buying a lot of new clothes, or using drugs, including alcohol. We're talking about doing good things for your body and your spirit. (For more on maintaining spiritual and physical wellness, see Chapters 12 and 13.)

Remember you're not alone. It's a time to be needy and get the need met. Here are some suggestions to help you keep yourself emotionally steady and focused on keeping your health at its best.

## MAXIMIZING YOUR HEALTH

1. *Get the support you need from family, counselors and support groups.*

Start by getting the support you need in order to stay on track. Take advantage of the counseling offered through your local AIDS advocacy organization or church. Keep your appointments with your drug or alcohol counselor. Open yourself up to family and friends who see the good in you, who believe in you, and spend time with these people.

Deciding whom to tell is often difficult. That's why finding help from others, even strangers, may give support that does not have any baggage associated with it. It is sometimes easier to talk to a stranger about something that is difficult—especially a stranger who is informed and associated with an organized support group, or with your clinic or local department of health, or with your church. Just be sure to check on the qualifications of anyone you do talk to. Most health care providers are very glad to answer questions about their training and reliability.

Telling people about your illness should not put you in danger. If there is a chance that the person you tell may react violently, talk to your health care provider, counselor or clergy for guidance. I notice that people who delay telling others for a long period often find, when they *do* finally tell, that their family and friends are fully supportive. Because these are the people closest to you, people with whom you share a common history, these people often provide the deepest support over long periods of time.

It is possible that some members of your family already suspect that you have HIV, or that you are gay, or that you have used drugs. Yet if yours is like many Black families, you have never spoken openly about it. Telling your family may be a big relief to everyone, allowing all of you to build a bond of trust. Even if you decide that you, or your family, aren't ready for the conversation, that doesn't mean that the story is closed. As time goes on, you may change your mind.

> *Telling your family may be a big relief to everyone, allowing all of you to build a bond of trust.*

You should strongly consider participating in a support group—especially right after you have received your test result. You are going to have a dialogue with yourself that is largely focused on issues that you cannot change and that only add to your stress. This is a time to get with people who have been through it too, not only to develop new relationships, but also to talk with those who have experience on the path you are now taking.

Being honest and open about HIV is especially important for Black Americans because of the destructive tendency of our community to be silent about the disease. You will be doing good for yourself and the community by attending a group in which you talk about your HIV. You will be helping to break the chain of silence and shame. Some of the sessions will be difficult, but with most you will feel rejuvenated.

If you are drawn to religion and spirituality, this is a time to reconnect to your spiritual side and gather the strength that comes from a church community (For more about spirituality and HIV, turn to Chapter 13.)

2. *Make it easy by being honest with yourself.*

Take a look at who you are and be honest with yourself about your own strengths and weaknesses. Taking stock means asking yourself questions. Here are some examples:

- Are you organized or disorganized—someone who often breaks appointments?
- Are you a planner or an impulsive person—for example, someone who has sex spontaneously?
- Do you have close family and friends or do you tend to feel isolated and alone?

In each case, you'll find that once you look at the truth about yourself you're on the way to making that truth work for you. For example, if you are generally a disorganized person, you may find it extra challenging to keep your medical appointments and to take your medications each day. Once you recognize the problem, you'll begin to see the solution.

The trick is to plan ahead. Develop a system that helps you remember your medications and appointments. Buy a small calendar or ask a friend to buy you one and put your appointments in it. Keep the calendar with you at all times. When you make appointments with the health care provider, ask if the office can call you the day before to remind you.

*Develop a system that helps you remember your medications and appointments.*

Ask the nurse to help you write out a chart of your medications and when they should be taken each day. Post the chart in your bedroom or kitchen. This is part of setting your life up so you can succeed. (For more about taking your medications, turn to Chapter 6.)

Remember that people who take all of their medication doses every day tend to have the highest CD4 counts and the lowest levels of virus in their blood streams. You can get there too if you stay organized! This principle can work in little things as well as in big ones—for example:

- If you tend to run out of cash for the bus that gets you to your appointments, buy a monthly bus pass. If you can't afford one, talk to the social worker at the clinic for assistance with paying.
- If you will need child care during your appointments, don't wait until the last minute to find someone. Talk to your family or baby-sitter now and schedule them well in advance.

- If you don't have someone who can do the extra child-care, see the social worker about other options.
- Look at your work schedule for the next few months. Will you need to take time off for medical or other appointments? If so, plan ahead to take sick days or personal days during that time.
- Get yourself some latex condoms and keep them handy—in your wallet, under your mattress. It's especially important to have condoms handy if you have unplanned sex. Buy them or get them free at your clinic.
- Do what you need to keep good food in the house, whether it's scheduling a once-a-week shopping trip, picking up your food stamps or asking the social worker to help you get money for a taxi or bus to get to the grocery store. (For more about good eating, see Chapter 12.)

Stress control is one of the most important things in your life to focus on. Learn to eliminate those aspects of your life that cause you the most stress and focus on changing them. Live within your means, don't get into debt, plan for expenses and put money away to cover them. Sometimes eliminating your extra credit cards or moving to less expensive housing can make a huge difference. In this case, stress control means finding a solution to a problem, instead of being paralyzed by it.

Try not to stress out! Staying relaxed is one of the most effective ways to keep your immune system strong. Regular exercise, such as walking for half an hour each day, taking time for yourself and, if it works for you, praying or meditating are just a few of the ways that people keep stress down. (Turn to Chapter 13 for more about stress and stress relief.)

*3. Create a professional relationship with your primary provider.*

The kind of relationship you have with your health care provider is vitally important. You will be seeing him or her at least every few months for years to come. The provider will get to know you very well.

If you have never before had a long-term and strong relationship with a primary provider, it may seem awkward to you. This person will know things about you that maybe even your significant other does not know. Do your part by giving honest answers to the questions he or she asks about your physical and emotional history. For example, if you used drugs in the past, the primary provider needs to know this. Don't worry. He or she is bound by oath to keep all identifying information about patients confidential.

*Do your part by giving honest answers to the questions your health care provider asks about your physical and emotional history.*

You should know that HIV health providers are among the smartest and most compassionate in the health field. You need to search hard to find a provider that you feel understands you as a patient and a person. Taking time to get a good match is worth the effort.

If you feel that you must change providers, do so. But before you do, be honest with your present provider about your feelings, even if what you tell the provider is that the relationship between you isn't working. This is nothing unusual so don't feel bad about it. It is important for you to feel good about your provider.

4. *Safe sex is a lifelong commitment to prevention.*

Make a promise to yourself and to the future of your community that you will only have safe sex. If you continue to have unsafe sex, you will infect others, and the HIV epidemic will continue. Expect to have sex; keep condoms with you. The guilt and stress that you should feel from having unsafe sex just isn't worth it.

Unsafe sex can also hurt you medically. It puts you in danger of contracting another population of HIV and may make your disease more challenging to treat. You have enough problems! Don't create more.

5. *Tell those you have exposed.*

Soon after you learn you are HIV-positive, the provider, nurse or caseworker will sit with you and help you determine when you may have become infected. The provider will also want to know whom you may have exposed to your HIV. Working back from the time you think you may have become infected, you will be asked to remember every person you had sex with or shared needles with. These people must be told that they are at risk for HIV/AIDS and need to get tested. You

---

*Make a promise to yourself and to the future of your community that you will only have safe sex. If you continue to have unsafe sex, you will infect others, and the HIV epidemic will continue.*

---

---

*Making sure that the people you have exposed to the HIV virus know they've been exposed is one of the most important things you can do to stop HIV from spreading in your community and to your friends.*

---

can tell them, or the clinic can do it for you without using your name.

Making sure that the people you have exposed to the HIV virus know they've been exposed is one of the most important things you can do to stop HIV from spreading in your community and to your friends. The practice of telling has helped many people with HIV learn early that they have the virus. Women with HIV have been able to start on medications to keep their babies from getting the disease, because somebody tipped the mothers off that they might be positive. You may allow both mother and baby to live longer and healthier by telling the mother she may have been infected by someone with HIV.

Naming those you may have infected can be a wrenching experience. You may feel ashamed, guilty and very angry about the entire situation. You may imagine that some of the people you tell will be furious at you and may cause you emotional pain. But you cannot turn back the clock and undo what you've done. None of us can. Thinking that you may have infected others will probably be one of the biggest regrets of your life. But having regrets is part of life. Make acting on them part of your life, too.

The healthiest way of dealing with regrets is not to blame yourself. It's better for others and for you, if you work to make the situation as right as possible—by letting people know they may have HIV, so they can get the medical treatment and the support they deserve. Let people you may have infected know, so they can get the medical treatment and the support they deserve. Giving the names of those people to your provider is another way of battling against this epidemic that threatens so many of us.

> *Let people you may have infected know, so they can get the medical treatment and the support they deserve.*

6. *You don't need money to get HIV/AIDS treatment.*

No person need go without treatment because of lack of money. All that's required is that you get your situation squared away. If you do not have health insurance, or if the insurance you have is not adequate to cover all your treatments, you still can receive the medical care you need. A federal law called the Ryan White Act, named for an HIV-positive boy who died of AIDS, provides free medical care for anyone with HIV who cannot afford to pay for treatment. This program includes money for drugs and living expenses.

> *A federal law called the Ryan White Act, named for an HIV-positive boy who died of AIDS, provides free medical care for anyone with HIV who cannot afford to pay for treatment. This program includes money for drugs and living expenses.*

Also, you may be eligible for veterans' benefits, Medicaid, Medicare, or special coverage through your state or AIDS advocacy organization. All the information you need is usually available at the HIV clinic, but if not, a call to your local or county health department will link you up to services.

*7. Do drug or alcohol detox.*

If you are an IV drug user, other drug user (illegal drugs or hormone injections), or drink heavily, you will be urged to go through detox and to stay substance-free. Any abusive practice wears your body down; this is especially so if you have HIV. Substance abuse will distract you from paying attention to your health needs and medication schedule, and it will make you get sick faster.

The caseworker or social worker can help you find a detox program. If you have tried in the past and haven't been able to quit, now is the time to try again and give it your all. Being free of addictions means having your life back. With today's AIDS drugs you have the chance to live well for many years. Why blow it all for the unsatisfying loneliness of addiction? (For more about HIV and drug abuse, see Chapter 11.)

# CHAPTER 5

# HIV-ITS PROGRESSION AND TREATMENT

One of the first challenges your health care provider faces in your case is to figure out what stage your HIV is in. The HIV moves through a number of phases, starting when you were infected, to the pre-disease period of about eight years, to HIV disease, and (in some people) to AIDS.

Determining the stage lets the provider and you know how much the virus has damaged your immune system. Even if you are healthy and without symptoms, "staging" helps your provider decide on your present treatment and the probable time when new developments are likely to occur. Of course, nobody knows for sure when you will have an opportunistic infection or will need to be put in the hospital, but by comparing your history of infections, your viral load and your CD4 count, your provider should be able to offer you some guidance.

Even if your CD4 count is very low, say 50, it is not too late to begin treatment. Most patients respond very well to the

*Even if your CD4 count is very low, say 50, it is not too late to begin treatment.*

start of antiretroviral drugs even when there are no detectable CD4 cells in their blood (late stage disease).

If your immune system is strong, you may not be given any treatment at this time. The reason health care providers wait (except for patients recently infected) before starting people on antiretroviral therapy is that the drugs are harsh and sometimes inconvenient to take. Once you start taking them, you must keep taking them for the rest of your life. Most experts agree that people should start taking antiretrovirals if their CD4 count is less than or equal to 350 on two separate tests. If you are having symptoms, you will be offered treatments aimed at your specific problem. Your body may, over time, build up a resistance to HIV drugs. (For more about antiretrovirals, turn to Chapter 6.)

By knowing something about the stages of HIV, you will be able to speak more easily with the provider about what you might expect, which will let you make plans and take back full control of your life.

## EARLY HIV DISEASE

We have talked about the Primary HIV Syndrome. Within a month or so of your being infected, the virus settles into your body for the long haul. It quietly moves into your cells and blood and stays there, giving few if any outward signs of disease, though it is detectable by clinical tests. As we discussed, though you will have few if any symptoms at this stage, you are infected with HIV and can pass the disease on to others.

This phase may last from three to fourteen years, depending on the characteristics of the virus itself, your immune response to it, and how well you take care of yourself. Follow the seven suggestions in "Maximizing Your Health" on pages 54–63 in Chapter 4. Take good care of yourself by eating balanced meals, getting good rest and exercise and avoiding stressful habits that may weaken your immune system.

Remember: although you may have no symptoms, the virus is attacking and killing cells and your body is fighting back by making new cells. This battle uses up an enormous amount of energy. That's why it's so important for you to develop good health habits now, and provide your body with the energy it needs to fight back.

While good physical health is essential, so is good mental health. Take time to relax and to enjoy yourself. Feeling relaxed and satisfied helps boost the immune system. This may sound absurd—you have a potentially fatal disease and we are telling you to relax. But I see it in my practice every day. Most people who begin and continue good medical care and support services live meaningful and satisfying lives, and you can, too.

*Most people who begin and continue good medical care and support services live meaningful and satisfying lives, and you can, too.*

Make sure the things that always gave you joy are still part of your daily life. Look for new activities that bring you joy and incorporate them into your routine. Such an activity might be any of the following:

- Attending church
- Walking outdoors
- Having meals with family and friends
- Going to clubs, parties or movies

All can be part of the healing process. When you are happy, and feel safe and loved, your immune system is healthier. (For more on keeping yourself well, turn to Chapter 12.)

If you are a drug or alcohol abuser and do not eat well, get stressed out and do not get a good night's sleep, the disease is likely to progress faster. Coke and crack will cause your CD4 count to drop more rapidly because of the lifestyle it brings when done over long periods of time.

If you are taking good care of yourself, your illness will progress more slowly. You will maintain a strong CD4 count and a low viral load (less than 10,000), and have no major outward symptoms of disease. If your CD4 counts are above 350 and you are not in an early stage of an infection, you may not be offered antiretroviral drugs by your provider. You must remember that even though you are early in the infection and haven't advanced to the point of needing ARV treatment, you can still infect others.

Changes usually take place gradually. But sometimes a CD4 count may drop suddenly and the virus will multiply quickly. This is especially likely to happen if you are heavily stressed, get an immunization, or if you get sick with a serious infection. It can also happen for no apparent reason.

Your health care provider's job becomes one of trying to keep your immune function at its highest level and anticipate the development of infections. This is why you need to contact him or her with any early symptoms of infection that you see or feel. The health care provider needs to get to know your illness and you. He or she tracks HIV progression by being alert to the symptoms of early infection, looking for signs to confirm, and monitoring the decline of immune function as reflected in the CD4 and viral load.

So it becomes critically important that you keep your appointments with your provider. The results of blood tests are likely to be the first signs, before you have symptoms, to show that your virus is starting to multiply, unchecked by your immune response. The sooner that is known, the sooner you can be given therapies to help limit viral growth and immune function destruction so you stay well.

If you start to experience symptoms of HIV and ignore them, you are giving the disease a chance to damage your immune system further. You will progress more rapidly to AIDS. Treatment can lower viral growth and markedly slow destruction of your immune function. You are worth the effort!

## HIV DISEASE

At some point, either you or your provider will notice that you aren't doing as well as you have in the past. You may feel more tired, or be getting more colds that are lasting longer, or having trouble with skin or other infections. When you go in for your checkup, your provider may tell you that your CD4 count has dropped or that your viral load has increased, and that your disease has progressed.

You may not feel any different as you enter later stages of HIV. But when your T-cells are at 350 or less, you may be offered antiretroviral drugs. If you are ready and the provider advises it, he or she will prescribe a variety of drugs for you that you will continue to take every day for the rest of your life. This is not easy, but don't be discouraged! The antiretroviral drugs available today offer you an opportunity not available to people with HIV disease ten years ago. Back then, people typically succumbed to the disease within two years of developing symptoms. Now, with the help of new drugs, many people are staying alive a long time with a diagnosis of AIDS. Nobody knows what future research may bring, but we trust it will bring more good news.

Here is what you can generally expect in Stage II (HIV disease) at various CD4 levels:

- If your CD4 count is above 500 and your viral load is between 10,000 and 20,000, you probably will have few if any symptoms of HIV infection. Your provider will probably tell you to focus on maintaining your health, and that you do not need to take antiretroviral drugs.
- If your CD4 count is 350 to 500 and your viral load has increased significantly, you may be offered the option of starting antiretroviral medications. The decision is up to you and your provider, and it depends on many factors, including how you are feeling. If you are not having any major symptoms of HIV disease, you may choose to wait.

Another reason for posibly waiting is that the provider wants to make sure that once the drugs are started, you will be able to take them as prescribed. If your life situation is such that it may be difficult for you to stick with a medication schedule, you may choose to wait until your situation changes. This is a time to aggressively rethink the factors in your life that are helping you and those that are not. Get help to think through what might be the best course of action. (For more about antiretrovirals, see Chapter 6.)

One factor important to consider is your viral load. If it is above 50,000, you may consider taking antiretrovirals. If it is above 10,000, your primary care provider may feel it is important to watch the viral load more closely for a few months. If the viral load is persistently elevated, your provider may suggest antiretroviral (ARV) therapy. The viral load does not seem to predict rates of progression as well as the CD4 count. Some experts rely more on the CD4 count in making decisions about starting ARV therapy.

- If your confirmed CD4 count is 350 to 500 and your viral load over 20,000, you may start having trouble with skin conditions, such as psoriasis, shingles and herpes. You may be more vulnerable to thrush, an overgrowth of yeast in the mouth, or to vaginal yeast infection, sinus infections and lung infections. You need to take extra precautions so as not to get infected with colds, flu and TB—precautions such as washing your hands *six* times a day and avoiding close contact with people you know are sick. Your provider may prescribe antibiotics or antifungal drugs to cure or prevent infections.

- If you're confirmed CD4 count drops below 350, even if you have no symptoms and regardless of your viral load, you will be offered antiretrovirals. The reason is that even if you aren't feeling bad, experience shows that starting ARVs will slow the decline of the CD4 count and prolong the time it takes for you to develop infections.

## AIDS

If your confirmed CD4 count is 200 or below, or if you develop an opportunistic infection or Kaposi's sarcoma, you are considered to have AIDS. Your provider will almost certainly prescribe antiretroviral medications of the type we describe below. These drugs will help boost your immune system, often to a CD4 count 130 units higher. So, if your CD4 count is 150, you might expect it to increase to 280 with medication.

At this stage, you are at great risk for opportunistic infections, diseases like Pneumocystis Carinii Pneumonia (PCP), a type of pneumonia, and toxoplasmosis, an infection of the

---

*At this stage, you are at great risk for opportunistic infections, diseases like Pneumocystis Carinii Pneumonia (PCP), a type of pneumonia, and toxoplasmosis, an infection of the brain that afflicts people whose immune systems are weakened.*

---

brain that afflicts people whose immune systems are weakened. You will be given antibiotics (trimethoprime sulfamethoxazole) to prevent PCP and toxoplasmosis. You may be given other medications as well.

Your primary provider will ask you to watch for symptoms like shortness of breath, cough or fever more than three days, or a new rash. These symptoms may mean you have an infection. (See more about opportunistic infections in Chapter 7.)

A secondary benefit of antiretrovirals is that if your CD4 goes above 200, it may be possible for you to stop taking the antibiotics and other drugs that prevent PCP and other diseases. Your own immune system, with a CD4 count above 200, will have enough fighting power to keep these diseases away from you.

When you start taking antiretrovirals, your immune system reconstitutes and fights hard against the opportunistic infections you have. As a result, your symptoms may worsen. The idea is that your immune system is getting itself back together so it can react to the invading infection. This causes a migration of white cells into the area where before there had been none, and this may create a flare of your symptoms. This is nothing to be alarmed about.

If your CD4 count drops to between 50 to 100, you will be vulnerable to Mycobacterium Avium Complex, or MAC, an atypical mycobacterium found in the soil. You may be offered a drug to prevent MAC infections. You are also prone to cytomegalovirus, or CMV, which we've described earlier.

If your CD4 count drops to less than 50, your immune system has diminished fighting power. The goal of your therapy is to try to prevent infection. This is done by taking:

- Trimethoprime sulfamethoxazole for PCP, bacterial pneumonia, and toxoplasmosis prevention, and
- Azithromycin for MAC prevention; untreated, you may have chronic diarrhea, which can lead to a wasting syndrome

You may feel weak some days with a low reserve.

Even at this late stage of illness, it has been clearly shown you too will benefit from ARV therapy. It is not too late—just more urgent that you get into care as soon as possible and begin to address the issues we have described. I have many patients who entered care with low or absent CD4 counts and who began treatment, started on ARVs, and showed dramatic recovery of their immune function and energy. Many have maintained a high quality of life for years.

# CHAPTER 6

# ANTIRETROVIRAL MEDICATIONS

Because your antiretroviral medications are such a critical part of living with HIV, you need to understand what these drugs are, how they work and how you can get them. In this chapter, you'll also learn something about the African Americans who fought to make these drugs available.

Antiretroviral drugs (ARVs) are drugs that fight HIV. They have been in use since the late 1980s, but a new, very effective group of these medications was discovered in the mid-1990s. These drugs have helped to change HIV infection from a disease that killed nearly everyone who had it, to a disease with which people could live for years. You may not believe this, but you're lucky to have gotten HIV at this time, when such effective therapy is available.

Take advantage of your luck. Don't be one of those African Americans who don't get diagnosed. Get on medication early enough to enjoy the greatest benefits of treatment.

Your health care provider will offer you antiretroviral drugs, typically, when your CD4 count is 350 or less, or your viral load is elevated to 55,000 or more if you are asymptomatic (for patients who are symptomatic a lower viral load may warrant initiation of therapy). You will also be offered antiretrovirals if, though your CD4 count is in a safe range, you are contracting opportunistic infections. Pregnant women also may take these drugs, even during pregnancy. (For more on pregnancy and HIV, see Chapter 9.)

*Take advantage of your luck. Don't be one of those African Americans who don't get diagnosed and on medication early enough to enjoy the greatest benefits of treatment.*

Taking three or more different antiretroviral drugs (a "cocktail") at one time is the most effective way to weaken the virus. Don't think you can take just one of the drugs and ignore the others. If you do that, the virus will develop a resistance to one or more of the drugs, and you will get sicker. (See pages 100–101 for more on drug resistance).

Providers and patients have seen amazing results with this therapy. The drug cocktails actually improve peoples' CD4 (increase) and viral load measurements (decrease), to the point where people feel much better, even healthy. It is not unusual that people who were too ill to work, run errands, or exercise are able to do so after taking these drugs. Their future opens up before them, and yours can, too.

## THE STRUGGLE FOR GOOD HEALTH CARE

These drugs, and these dramatic recoveries, are possible largely because people with HIV demanded better medical treatment.

Family and friends, and just plain sympathetic people, many of whom had lost friends, fought alongside those with HIV. Some people fought simply out of a sense of justice. It was a powerful coalition, of the sick and the well, the straight and the gay. It showed that medical issues could be addressed as civil rights issues. Certainly the benefits of this struggle were great. Today all Americans with HIV can enjoy them.

How it worked was this: HIV/AIDS concerned groups spoke to the U.S. Congress and wrote letters to the President. They demonstrated at scientific conferences, and spent a lot of time trying to convince those who control research money in this country to spend more of it on HIV research. Their efforts paid off when much more money was given to HIV research, treatment and prevention programs.

What the story shows is that the struggle for better health care is today's version of the civil rights movement. Nothing is more important to our community than that we take action for better health care. Action begins by learning more about what makes us healthy and what makes us ill, and how to get the best treatment available. It also means looking at ourselves, and asking hard questions about why we African Americans, as individuals and as a group, don't go after the good health care that's readily available to us. What is it about our psychic makeup that prefers to endure extraordinary symptoms, before we go to the clinic or emergency room? Why, for so many diseases (HIV included) do we, as a group, enter treatment late and have higher rates of suffering and death? And why have we been slow to learn, as individuals and as a community, the diets and behaviors that make us strong and well, along with those that make us sick and weak?

Today, the Black community is mobilizing to address the needs presented to them by HIV. African American individuals, including Dr. Benny Primm, Dr. David Satcher, Dr. Helen Gayle, Ms. Fredette West, Mr. Phil Wilson and Mr. Cornelius Baker have joined institutions and organizations that include the CBC (Congressional Black Caucus), DHHS (Department of Health and Human Services), the Black Church, the Balm in Gilead, Black Leadership Commission on AIDS, the African American AIDS Policy and Training Institute and many others, to create the Minority AIDS Initiative.

This Initiative helped create a federal funding line to support research and educational programs focused on the unmet needs of the African American HIV-infected community. Hundreds of millions of dollars now flow into Black American communities. The money supports expansion in HIV-related prevention and treatment programs.

Of course there's also bad news. The money hasn't been enough and requires renewal every year with a new budget. So the struggle goes on. By raising your voice against the injustice (sometimes called "the death gap") that causes Black people to get poorer medical treatment than White People, you can be part of the struggle to improve the health of our community.

Sure, there's injustice. But we can start pushing back against it by educating ourselves on the issues. In that way we enter the fight. It all starts with you. By seeing your health care provider regularly, taking your medication, eating well and getting exercise, you're making a statement. You're saying, I take responsibility for my own health, I value my life, and I value the life of the community. (To learn more about the

Minority Aids Initiative and other resources available to you, see the Resources section at the end of this book.)

## PAYING FOR YOUR DRUGS

In the United States, every person is entitled to treatment with antiretroviral drugs when that treatment is appropriate. If money is an issue for you, the federal government will pay for your care and drugs through the Ryan White CARE Act. This program created free treatment service in all fifty states and fifty-two cities that are especially hard hit by HIV. Contact your local Department of Health for referral sites near you. If you need help paying for medications, tell your primary care provider or social worker, who can help set you up with a program to help you. (For more about how to find assistance to pay for HIV medications, see the Resources section at the end of this book.)

> *If money is an issue for you, the federal government will pay for your care and drugs through the Ryan White CARE Act.*

## THE DRUGS WORK IN EVERYONE

If you have heard that AIDS drugs work only in White people, don't believe it. Like aspirin, cough syrup and other drugs, these drugs work in all people. Yes, a drug's ability to work is affected by ones' genetic make up, but race does not play an important part in the effectiveness of the antiretrovirals. That has been proven in tests that include Black Americans. I have treated hundreds of African Americans with these drugs, the vast majority of whom have done very well. Thousands of Black people are on these drugs now, and doing well because of them. So don't believe the street rumors. By not taking these drugs, some Black people are keeping themselves from the best therapies available—therapies that everyone else is taking and benefiting from. It is time that Black people benefit, too.

In people who take these drugs, the progression from HIV to AIDS is slowed, and opportunistic infections are more rare and less severe. Most of these people have regained their energy and created hope for the future. They are truly living with HIV. As one person with HIV recently told me, describing himself and his friends, "We are taking out long-term loans again, and applying for long-term mortgages."

Yes, there are problems with the drugs: they can have strong side effects, and it is a hassle to take so many pills every single day. But the drugs make most people better. They extend the lives of the people who take them correctly and take good care of themselves. In the meantime, we're working to reduce the side effects and to simplify the dosages.

## EXPERIMENTAL DRUGS

New HIV drugs are constantly under study and being tested on people in clinical drug trials. If you are interested in taking part, find out all you can about the drug from your local AIDS advocacy group, or your HIV clinic. (In the Resources section at the end of this book, see the section on AIDS Clinical Trials Group (ACTG) for more information.)

You are under no obligation to join these studies of new drugs. In fact, the health care provider must ask YOUR permission to give you an experimental drug or for you to be enrolled in a clinical trial of a drug.

Experimental drugs are recommended when people have not responded to, or no longer respond to, already available drugs. Most African Americans have not been on and off of therapy, and, as a result, have not "used up" the ability for any one drug to kill HIV. So for most of us, the tried and true drugs, the ones that have been proven safe and effective, are still effective.

The fear among African Americans of being experimented on is a real fear. If your health care provider has recommended that you take experimental drugs and you feel mistrust, tell him or her that you are afraid of being taken advantage of or experimented on. Make sure the provider knows how you feel, and is willing to explain why he or she thinks these drugs are best for you. The provider may be part of a team doing research for a new drug. Ask about that. Even if it is the case, the drug may still be the best drug for you. Whether or not the provider persuades you that this drug represents the best treatment, you'll better understand your treatment options.

The trick is to take your time and to ask questions until you are satisfied that you know everything you need to know. You may want to ask questions like these:

- How long have the drugs been in use and what are their side effects (short-term and long-term)?
- Why has the health care provider chosen the particular combination he or she is offering you?

- What benefits can you expect from this particular treatment?
- How does the drug combination you are offered affect your drug choices in the future?

Most HIV health care providers know the sad history that makes African Americans suspicious of the medical establishment. They will welcome your questions, and you will be well on your way to the communicative and cooperative relationship with your provider that will best serve your health interests.

## HAVE A PLAN FOR WHEN TO START ANTIRETROVIRAL THERAPY

*If your CD4 count is not strong and you are not feeling well, you take a big risk by not starting on therapy*

If you do not take drugs, at some point you will surely get sicker, so don't "blow off" the decision whether to begin. If your CD4 count is not strong and you are not feeling well, you take a big risk by not starting on therapy. (See Chapter 7 for more on opportunistic infections.)

Granted, things may be going on in your life that make it necessary to delay treatment, just for the time it takes to get that specific problem resolved. Maybe you've just become pregnant and want to wait until the first trimester (four months) is over, to protect the baby. During the first trimester brain development is critical, and although we have not seen problems with the fetus, doctors often wait until this period is over before starting any drugs, including antiretrovirals.

Other kinds of problems too can bear on your decision to start treatment. Maybe you're about to move into a new apartment and need some time to get settled. Maybe you're working to kick a habit of substance abuse, or just to get yourself into a more stable living situation.

So talk over with your health care provider when is the best time for you to begin, carefully examining the advantages and disadvantages of delay. Remember, delay now may mean that you will need different and stronger treatment when you do begin.

As you plan with your provider the time to begin treatment, you'll also want to talk about early symptoms of an opportunistic infection. That kind of discussion will help you recognize such an infection early.

The bottom line is that if you don't take these drugs, your CD4 count will drop and you will get sick. If you don't get treated and then develop AIDS, treatment can be more of a problem. On average, people diagnosed with AIDS who do not take any drugs at all die within three years. Their CD4 count on average will drop by about 80 points each year. Starting with a CD4 count of 300, someone who didn't take the drugs would have a CD4 count of less than 200 within two years, and less than 100 two years later. This person's ability to stay alive and well at that rate would be uncertain.

*On average, people diagnosed with AIDS who do not take any drugs at all die within three years.*

Sadly, the majority of people who live with HIV are in China, India and the sub-Sahara, where drugs are not easily available or are too expensive for them. You have the privilege of living in a country where the drugs are available. Don't waste that privilege.

## PREPARING FOR ANTIRETROVIRAL THERAPY

Before you start on antiretroviral therapy, set up your life to make it easy for you to keep taking the drugs even if you have side effects. You should be prepared to feel bad for three to four weeks when you begin the medications. This happens to *everyone.* You are adjusting to these powerful medications as they kill hundreds of thousands of virus particles. In nearly everyone, during the first month, this causes some nausea, vomiting, diarrhea, mild abdominal discomfort, low-grade fever, increased sweating and variable fatigue.

Don't let the side effects defeat you. Don't even think of stopping your drugs until you have gone through four weeks on therapy. You'll get through this tough period easily if you follow the example of others before you: talk to your health care provider and to a friend who has been through this. Get involved with support groups. We do better with struggles like this when we have the emotional support of others behind us.

*Don't let the side-effects defeat you.*

Keep focused on the fact that you will feel better once your body gets used to the drugs, and that all these early symptoms go away forever. But if you start and stop your medications, you'll have to go through this start up phase again and again. This is a critical point to remember. Everyone must go through this difficult period of getting used to the medications. Don't be discouraged by it.

If you can, plan to start the drugs at a time when you have a light workload, your child is in school during the day, or child care will be easily available if you do not feel well. Ideally, begin the drugs when you will have some support available. Tell a close friend to be on "alert" in case you need him or her to take care of you for a few days, for grocery shopping or other errands.

*It's important that you be in a position to take all the drugs once you start them and to take them correctly.* You will have to work closely with your pharmacist and health care provider to make sure that you keep a steady supply of medications in your house. You need to keep track of when your medication supply is getting low and make sure to get the prescriptions refilled. When you get your prescriptions filled, choose a pharmacy that is close to your home or where you work, one that is easy to get to. Always refill your prescriptions at this same pharmacy. That way, the pharmacist has the opportunity to get to know you and any special concerns you may have about the drugs, such as allergies or side effects, or drug interaction with new medications.

*You need to keep track of when your medication supply is getting low and make sure to get the prescriptions refilled.*

The pharmacist is a good person to talk to about your medications. He or she has real expertise about how they interact with each other and how best to take them. The pharmacist also knows about side effects, and can remind you what to be on the look out for in the way of early symptoms, and what you can do to live more comfortably with them. If you are worried about privacy, you can have this conversation on the phone anonymously.

When you pick up your drugs from the pharmacist, find out when they must be refilled and write this date on the bottle. *Don't run out of your drugs!* Refill them the week before they are due to run out. It is also helpful to put your medicines where you can find them. That may mean in your medicine cabinet or glove compartment or office. Keep a few extra doses set aside in the same place, in case you get caught short. (See more on pill management under "Organizing Your Medications," page 90–93.)

### WHY A DRUG COCKTAIL?

Each of the three classes of antiretroviral drugs works in slightly different ways to attack the virus. The drugs you take—your cocktail—may be drawn from any of the three classes or from one single class. Your health care provider makes this decision on the basis of your antiretroviral history, the stage of disease you are in, and whatever can be inferred from the virus you are infected with (resistance patterns).

Your provider may try a combination of drugs for a few months and then need to change it because it is not working out well for you. This does not mean the drugs are bad. They simply work differently in different people. It may take one or two tries to figure out which cocktail is the ideal one for you. It is important for you to be patient.

There are a couple of reasons that the drugs are given in combination. One is that the many different populations of the HIV virus have different patterns of resistance to particular drugs. Many people have more than one population of HIV. You may have one or more of the resistant types. Some drugs work best on certain populations. Others don't work well at all. Taking more than one drug gives you a better chance of successfully attacking each population of the virus you have, and getting your viral load down as quickly as possible. *In short, it is harder for the virus to develop resistance to the medications if they are given in combination than if they are given one at a time.*

Because each class of drug attacks the virus in a different way, a cocktail launches an attack on several fronts, which makes the virus unable to reproduce itself. This is reflected in a drop in your viral load, the goal being to reach the "undetectable" status. Within one week there will be clear laboratory evidence that your viral load is dropping, but the viral load won't reach its steady state for about three months.

## THE IMPORTANCE OF COMPLIANCE

Good compliance means taking the medications as they were prescribed. You will be taking many pills a day for two to four weeks. You will experience the symptoms we outlined above. But you absolutely must take them as prescribed. If you do not, the drugs will not work well and your health will deteriorate. If you miss taking a dose, within hours the virus will be multiplying rapidly again. You'll have given the virus just the opportunity it is waiting for to regain ground in its fight for your body.

The reason your regular doses are necessary is that antiretrovirals are not like other drugs. They are just strong enough to keep ahead of the virus. That's why a missed dose can be a critical setback to your health. People who take all the doses get stronger and do well. Although people who miss doses but stay on medication do better then those not taking any ARV medications, the chance of their having continued viral production (replication) goes way up.

If you are thinking about stopping the medications, you must talk with your provider *before* stopping the drugs. *If you must stop the drugs, never stop just one or two—stop all the ARV drugs at the same time.* This will prevent the premature development of resistance. (For more on this subject, see "Resistance," on pages 100–101.)

> *Never stop just one or two— stop all the ARV drugs at the same time.*

The key point is that it's greatly to your advantage to stay on the medications. One recent study found that people who took their medicine in the correct way 95 percent of the time had great success suppressing the virus. They often had no detectable virus in their blood. People who took their medicine in the correct way about 70 percent of the time had much more virus in their blood, and more virus means more rapid progression towards an AIDS defining opportunistic infection.

There's still another reason that not taking your medications as prescribed is playing with fire. The viruses in you develop resistance to the drug—that is, they learn to live in the presence of the drug. The worst-case scenario on this is that a strain of virus resistant to every drug available *could* develop. It hasn't happened yet, and by taking your medications as prescribed, you're helping to prevent this situation from developing.

People who are organized and find it easy to live by schedules have an easier time following the necessary pill-taking schedule. But even for well-organized people, the new responsibility and emotional strain of taking care of oneself, added to all the old problems, can make it hard to keep the routine. That's why we strongly recommend that if you haven't done so already, link up with an HIV support group. People in the group will be going through what you are, and hearing how they worked out their problems can help you handle the stress. And who knows, you just may be able to offer some advice or support to someone else.

If you are struggling with drug addiction, alcohol abuse or depression, it may be harder for you to believe that things can change, that your life can get better, or even that you are worth the effort. You most definitely are! You're a human being and human life is too precious to be thrown away carelessly.

So take a deep breath, then take a long hard look at your life. Particularly, face up to the things that are causing you stress—including addictions. By dealing with the problem, you stay in touch with your sense of your own self-worth. When your addictions are under control your whole life goes better, and you're better able to manage the schedule of medications that can make you well. When you are using, things fall apart.

If you find yourself getting stressed by the challenge of scheduling your HIV drugs, get counseling, as a way of committing yourself to turning away from drugs or alcohol. Anyway, you need someone to talk to who can help you handle the stress of taking your medicine regularly, staying off drugs and dealing with all the daily issues of your life. So get help, and don't wait until things fall apart.

Keep in mind that there just isn't much slack. Your body needs your full attention. Watch for the signs that mean you are stressing out, and then make sure you have a plan to respond to the stress and manage it quickly. Your counselor can help you develop your resources for managing stress. Talk to your counselor or provider whenever you feel you might be headed toward trouble. The earlier you spot the trouble and make the call, the better chance you have of stopping the trouble before it gets into high gear.

If because of some emergency you have to stop taking a drug, talk with your health care provider first. Your provider may be able to prescribe an alternative or give you information to help you better tolerate the problem drug. That way, your treatment won't suffer a major setback. If your provider agrees that you need to stop taking the drugs, be sure to stop them all at once, to avoid developing drug-resistance to the virus.

*It is reckless to decide to stop your cocktail on your own, without careful medical consultation.*

It is reckless to decide to stop your cocktail on your own, without careful medical consultation.

## ORGANIZING YOUR MEDICATIONS

When you begin antiretroviral therapy, you may have to take ten or more pills three times a day. In addition to the antiretroviral drugs, you may be on drugs to help you fight infections, and other drugs to help control side effects of the other ones. You may also take vitamins. All that can add up to twenty or more pills, three times a day!

Remember your pill schedule. First, sit down with the nurse and come up with a schedule that will work well for you. There is always flexibility. The nurse knows that if you have a schedule that makes sense to you, you're more likely to keep it. You can also adjust a schedule you've tried but found not practical. In such a case, talk to the nurse about adjusting it.

Here's an example of the kind of scheduling detail you may have to work out. Say one drug you have been given needs to be taken on an empty stomach three times a day, and the nurse has suggested you take it at 8 A.M., 1 P.M. and 8 P.M. But you usually eat your breakfast at 8 A.M. Don't change your mealtime unless you absolutely have to. Instead, take your pill at 7A.M., 2 P.M. and 9 P.M.. Come up with a schedule that suits your life.

Take your pills at the same time each day. That will make it easier for you to remember and for the pill-taking to become routine. Also, your body will become accustomed to receiving the pills at that time.

The pills must be taken in the correct dose. Some drugs are taken with food, some on an empty stomach. If you are not generally an organized person, the nurse can help you learn to be. She will probably give you a pillbox for pill taking. Use the pillbox! Don't try to remember everything. That is too much to expect of yourself.

If you did not get a pillbox and you think you need one, call the nurse and ask for one. If your clinic does not have one, get one from your local HIV or AIDS organization. The pillbox lists all your pills and the times of day when they need to be taken. This makes it easier to see when you should take which pill. Make a pill list and schedule to carry around, and put up other lists in places that will remind you what to take and when to take it.

On your regular calendar, note the day that your pills will run out. Then, go back one week and mark that day clearly. That is when you should go to the pharmacist to refill your pills.

Ask the provider or the friend who is with you to write down any special instructions for taking your pills, including food-related directions and storage issues. Again, don't try to remember this. Most people forget as soon as they leave the provider's office. If you realize later that you have forgotten the directions or don't understand them, ask the pharmacist to explain them to you or call your clinic.

Almost all the drugs have some side effects. If the provider doesn't mention them, that means he or she forgot. Ask about any possible side effects and what you should do to relieve them. This way you know what to expect, so there's less stress. (Your pharmacist can also review with you the possible side effects of your drugs.)

After you get your pills from the pharmacy, bring them home and immediately remove a one-week supply of each drug. Set this "stash" aside, perhaps in the refrigerator. If your pills need to be refrigerated and you don't have a reliable refrigerator, get a new one, or perhaps buy or borrow a mini-refrigerator.

If you run out of your pills at some point and cannot replace them immediately, you won't have to miss any doses; you can tap your stash. If possible, keep a smaller supply of pills (one-two doses) in the glove compartment of your car and in a safe place at work.

Keep your pills in the same place, like a kitchen cabinet or a night table by your bed or in the bathroom, so you see them every day and you don't have to hunt around for them. This is vitally impor-

> *Take your pills at the same time each day.*

tant in case of an emergency. If you keep your pills in a particular place you can tell someone else, your family or a friend, where to find them in an emergency.

People use to a lot of different tricks to remember to take their pills. You can write the times in your daily calendar or hand-held computer organizer. If you prefer, set the alarm on your watch to go off at the time that you need to take your pills.

Link taking your pills with something else you do, like brushing your teeth. Take your morning and evening pills before you brush your teeth.

## GET SUPPORT

If you haven't already, this is a good time to join a support group or group counseling session for HIV-positive people. You may get tips from other people about how to handle antiretrovirals and their side effects, and you will be offered support from others who have lived through what you are going through. Please don't keep your troubles to yourself. By opening up a little to others you may find you become happier and stronger.

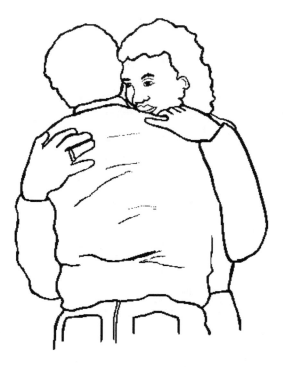

Don't forget, many, many other people have gone through what you are going through now. It may seem impossible to imagine, but some of these people had bigger challenges in their lives than you and they struggled through. If they did it, so can you!

For a while, it may feel like the antiretroviral drugs rule your entire life.

But over time, you will adjust. The pill taking will become routine and you won't have to think about it as you do now. It may never feel "normal," but you will not have to think about it every day, as you do now.

*Please don't keep your troubles to yourself. By opening up a little to others you may find you become happier and stronger.*

Maybe you've never stuck to a program in the past. But that was then, this is now. We can all change, especially when so much is at stake for our loved ones and ourselves.

## FOOD

You may have to make adjustments in your diet when you begin taking antiretroviral drugs. You may have to change your meal times, for instance, because some drugs are best taken on an empty stomach, others with a fatty meal. You may have to start eating certain foods, like yogurt, to help your digestive tract, or to avoid other foods that interact with the drugs you are taking. (For suggestions about how to make these changes, see Chapter 12.)

## BENEFITS YOU CAN EXPECT FROM ANTIRETROVIRALS

Within about a month of starting anti-retrovirals, your symptoms will decrease and you will begin to feel better. You will see a gradual decrease in fatigue. You will feel better and stronger because the drugs are raising your CD4 count—potentially, by 130 points or even more. So, if your CD4 count is 300 when you begin the drugs, over time it may increase to 420 or more. This means you have more active immune cells in your body to fight off opportunistic infections and HIV.

*Within about a month of starting antiretrovirals, your symptoms will decrease and you will begin to feel better. You will see a gradual decrease in fatigue.*

Another big benefit you'll experience when you get on regular medication is that you become less vulnerable to infections. If your CD4 count gets high enough, meaning your immune system is strong and functioning, your provider may suggest that you stop taking some of the antibiotics and other drugs that have helped you fight infections. When your immune system is strong, you won't need them.

With drug therapy, your immune system will strengthen and the number of virus particles in your blood (the viral load) will go down. Usually, and especially in patients who have never taken antiretroviral drugs before, the virus is undetectable in the blood. This doesn't mean the virus is gone, unfortunately. It means there are so few particles that testing can't pick them up. The virus continues to live inside you, in places the drugs can't reach, such as your lymph nodes, bone marrow, liver, spleen, eyes and brain. Here, the virus continues to multiply at a very slow rate. There is no test to count the number of virus particles outside of the blood.

Between two and eight weeks after you begin taking antiretrovirals, your health care provider will want you to have a checkup, to make sure the drugs are working correctly and that you are not in any danger from their side effects. The clinic will examine your CD4 and viral load counts and may also look for warning signs of serious drug side effects, such as liver or other problems.

Your primary care provider can tell as soon as one week after you start taking the drugs if they are working as intended. At three months, your virus may be undetectable. But if after a week you are not responding, you need to be switched to different drugs.

As early as one week after starting drug therapy, you should see a 20% drop in viral load. Recent data shows that if that you don't see this drop in a week, you will not completely suppress replication to "undetectable." Waiting too much longer than one week to make a change in drugs is not a good idea, as it gives the virus a chance to multiply unchecked and may increase the chance of developing resistance.

The provider will ask you about any side effects you are having and may offer suggestions as to how to cope with them. You will be asked to return to the clinic at least every three or four months to monitor the drugs you are taking and your response to therapy. You must hang in there, especially in the first few weeks after starting the drugs. The drugs *can* be tailored to suit your body, but this can only be done in a trial and error fashion over time, orchestrated by you and your provider.

## SIDE EFFECTS

Because these drugs are powerful, they can produce unwanted side effects along with their benefits. Some of the side effects are severe, such as stomach upset, bad diarrhea or numbness in your hands and feet. See your provider if you develop rashes, especially when you start taking a new drug. Other severe symptoms may include blood in your urine or stool, muscle aches or constant nausea. With some drugs, especially with Crixivan®, it is critical to increase your daily water intake.

The side effects may last for four weeks. In most people, they begin to go away after that, as the body adjusts to the drug. Some people want to give up when they experience these early side effects, because they feel so terrible. You may feel this way and, no way around it, those few weeks can be an awful experience. It takes sheer commitment on your part to trust that you will feel better, both from the side effects and from the HIV, after your body adjusts to the drugs. This is a big challenge that millions of people have met with flying colors, simply because they wanted to live.

Feeling that you can call your health care provider freely whenever you have a problem or stress about the medication is especially critical during the first few weeks of starting a new drug combination. You need to always be clear on what to expect from each drug and to be mindful of when a side effect is too severe to endure. Staying in close touch with your provider and support groups will help you handle that.

In addition to short-term side effects, there can be serious long-term effects that develop over time, including:

- Diabetes
- Liver enlargement
- Fatty liver
- Fat redistribution
- Kidney stones
- Lactic acidosis

Your health care provider will check you regularly for signs of these side effects, depending on the specific drug you are taking. There are treatments for some of the side effects. We mention some below.

Your provider or pharmacist has probably talked with you already about the side effects of your antiretroviral medications. If you are very uncomfortable from the side effects and for some reason can't reach your provider or talk to your pharmacist, go to the emergency room for help. Don't suffer needlessly!

If you can't get yourself to the emergency room and have no one to take you there, call your local HIV/AIDS advocacy organization. People there may be able to suggest over-the-counter remedies and offer you support until you hook up with your provider.

Don't be like Anita, who says, "I don't want to be any trouble," and "I don't want to deal with that medical establishment." The health care system is there to serve you, and you've never needed it more than you do now. Be aggressive about getting the help you need when you need it.

In some cases, side effects may be so severe and troublesome that your provider may have to switch you to a different drug. This doesn't mean that the first drug wasn't doing its job, only that your body couldn't tolerate the side effect. A drug failure means that your viral load increases in the presence of the drug. In such a case, your provider will eliminate that drug, and, possibly, other drugs in the same class, from your treatment.

Remember that you are not alone. Thousands of people are going through the same thing. They have hung in there for the great reward of continuing life—and so can you.

## RESISTANCE

A reason for the cocktail therapy is that over time, some populations of the virus have become resistant to certain drugs. A major reason this has happened is that people did not take the drugs as prescribed. They stopped one or two drugs while continuing the third, or took fewer doses. The virus learned how to overcome the drugs and went on dividing and attacking white cells and weakening the immune system, resulting in more rapid progression of the disease.

Once the virus became resistant to a certain drug, people spread this resistant virus to other people by having unprotected sex with them or by sharing needles.

These people in turn passed it on in the same way. This kind of behavior feeds the epidemic.

Even if you develop a resistant strain of HIV, don't panic. Fortunately, there are different combinations of drugs to try. Your health care provider will determine which drug isn't working, take you off of it, and replace it with a different drug. With drug cocktails, there is a good chance that, even if the virus is resistant to one drug in the cocktail, the others still control the virus and keep it from multiplying.

## RESISTANCE TESTING

Sometimes drug resistance develops for no known reason. In other cases, a person with HIV, by having unsafe sex or sharing needles, will pick up a new population of virus, and the drugs stop working. This resistance can be detected with genotypic or phenotpyic resistance testing. These are expensive tests that are widely used but poorly understood.

The genotypic testing looks for actual portions of the viral RNA that we know are associated with resistance to specific antiretrovirals. This method actually looks at the RNA sequences associated with known resistance.

The phenotypic method takes the virus in a person and sees if it can grow (replicate) in the presence of different anti-retrovirals.

Using both tests, your health care provider can profile your resistance pattern(s), and, in most instances, come up with a regimen that will work for you. In other words, if you prove to have resistance to one of these drugs, your provider will switch you to another drug or combination of drugs. Of course, if you skip having your scheduled blood work done, there is no way for your provider to know there is a problem.

## DRUG TOXICITY

Occasionally, people who have been taking drugs for a while begin to have a hard time handling them. Especially in some-one with a weak liver or kidneys, the drugs build up in the body and make the person feel sick. If this happens to you, your provider may switch you to new medications or may take you off of medication altogether for a short period so your body can clear the drugs that have built up.

Other long-term side effects happen, too. These include problems that can cause heart disease, such as high blood lipids (cholesterol and triglycerides), development of ele-vated blood sugar (diabetes), lactic acidosis (see "Long-Term Side Effects" on pages 111–112), and abnormal distribution of fat (lipodystrophy).

# MEDICATIONS AND SIDE EFFECTS

### Nucleoside transcriptase inhibitors (nukes)

These drugs prevent the viral RNA from changing into DNA, by the use of an enzyme found in the cytoplasm of your host cells called "reverse transcriptase enzyme." These drugs all have been associated with the development of a condition called Lactic Acidosis and severe liver problems, which are relatively rare but serious side effects. Specific drugs will have specific additional side effects. These drugs include:

- Abacavir (Ziagen; Trizivir): About 5% of patients will have a serious allergic reaction that may cause death if the drug is not stopped right away. Signs of this serious reaction include a skin rash or one or more of these symptoms: fever; nausea, vomiting, diarrhea, abdominal (stomach) pain; extreme tiredness, achiness, generally ill feeling; sore throat, shortness of breath, cough.

  Other side effects with Abacavir are nausea, vomiting, feeling generally ill or tired, headache, diarrhea, loss of appetite and changes in body fat.

- Didanosine (DDI) may cause peripheral neuropathy (a problem with the nerves in your hands or feet); inflamed pancreas, a serious side effect; and changes in vision. Other side effects with DDI are diarrhea, neuropathy, chills or fever, rash, abdominal pain, weakness, headache and nausea and vomiting.

- Lamivudine (3TC; Epivir). Children with a history of prior anti-retroviral nucleoside exposure, pancreatitis or other significant risk factors for the development of pancreatitis should use this medication with caution. Fat redistribution may also occur.

  Other adverse reactions may include nausea and vomiting, diarrhea, anorexia and/or decreased appetite, stomach upset (pain, cramp and indigestion), dizziness, fatigue and/ or malaise, headache, fever or chills, dreams, insomnia and other sleep disorders, and skin rash, problems with nerves, depression, cough, nasal problems, muscle pain and joint pain.

- Stavudine (D4T; Zerit) may cause nerve damage of the hands and feet (peripheral neuropathy), and pancreatitis (inflammation of the pancreas, which may result in stomach pain, nausea or vomiting),. Other side effects may include headache, diarrhea, rash, nausea and vomiting, stomach pain, muscle pain, insomnia, loss of appetite, chills or fever, allergic reactions and blood disorders.

- Trizivir. combination of AZT, 3TC and Abacavir. See each drug for side effect profile. Trizivir can also cause dizziness and pain or tingling in your hands or feet.

- Zalcitabine (DDC; Hivid) may cause severe peripheral neuropathy (tingling in arms and legs), particularly in those patients with advanced cases of the disease. It may also cause pancreatitis and hepatic failure (which may be fatal). Other serious side effects may include oral ulcers, stomach ulcers, heart failure, changes in body fat, and allergic reaction.

· Zidovudine (Retrovir, previously known as AZT), may cause bone marrow suppression, blood disorders (severe anemia and low levels of blood cells) and muscle weakness. Other side effects may include nausea, vomiting, weakness, headache, generally feeling ill, anorexia, constipation, stomach upset (pain, cramp and indigestion), joint pain, chills, feeling tired, elevated liver enzymes, trouble sleeping, muscle and joint pain and neuropathy (nervous system disorder).

### *Nucleotide Reverse Transcriptase Inhibitors*
· Tenofovir (Viread) may cause diarrhea, nausea, vomiting and intestinal gas. Other less common side effects may include weakness, inflammation of the pancreas, low blood phosphate, dizziness, shortness of breath and rash. Some patients have developed kidney problems. In some cases of patients taking anti-HIV medicine, body fat changes have also been seen.

### *Non-nucleoside Transcriptase Inhibitors (NNRTIs)*
These drugs work in a way similar to nukes above. NNRTIs include:

· Delavirdine mesylate (Rescriptor) may cause a skin rash on the upper body and upper arms, sometimes on the neck and face. The rash usually appears as a red area on the skin with slight bumps; it may be itchy. Other side effects may include headache, nausea, diarrhea and tiredness.

- Efavirenz (Stocrin; Sustiva): A small number of patients experience severe depression, strange thoughts, angry behavior, thoughts of suicide and, very rarely, actual suicide. Other side effects include dizziness, trouble sleeping, drowsiness, trouble concentrating and/or unusual dreams, rash, tiredness, upset stomach, vomiting and diarrhea and changes in body fat.

- Nevirapine (Viramune) may cause a severe rash and hepatitis. In rare cases, liver problems led to liver failure, which can lead to liver transplants or death. Other side effects include changes in body fat.

### Protease Inhibitors

Protease Inhibitors are very powerful in killing the virus in combination with NRT and NNRTIs. They work by blocking the enzyme protease, which is used to assemble the virus in the cytoplasm of the host cell. All the protease inhibitors have been associated with increased bleeding in patients with hemophilia, GI intolerance, elevated glucose and increases in cholesterol, triglycerides and body fat redistribution.

These drugs, with their side effects, include:

- Amprenavir ( Agenerase) may cause a severe rash. Other side effects may include diarrhea, nausea and vomiting, a tingling feeling, especially around the mouth, and change in taste. These effects are usually mild to moderate. Other reported side effects include depression and mood problems, changes in body fat, seizures, drowsiness, fast heart rate and kidney and blood abnormalities. Other side effects may include high blood sugar or diabetes, diabetes complications, high cholesterol or high triglycerides.

· Indinavir ( Crixivan): Some patients treated with Crixivan developed kidney stones. In some of these patients, development of kidney stones leads to more severe kidney problems, including kidney failure or inflammation of the kidneys, or kidney infection that sometimes spreads to the blood.

Some patients treated with Crixivan have had rapid breakdown of red blood cells (hemolytic anemia) which in some cases was severe or resulted in death. Some patients treated with Crixivan also have had liver problems including liver failure and death.

Other side effects include diabetes and high blood sugar, increased bleeding in patients with hemophilia, severe muscle pain and weakness, changes in body fat, increased liver enzymes, abdominal pain, fatigue or weakness, low red blood cell count, flank pain, painful urination, feeling unwell, nausea, upset stomach, diarrhea, vomiting, acid regurgitation, increased or decreased appetite, back pain, headache, dizziness, taste changes, rash, itchy skin, yellowing of the skin and/or eyes, upper respiratory infection, dry skin, sore throat, swollen kidneys due to blocked urine, allergic reactions, severe skin reactions, heart problems including heart attack, stroke, abdominal swelling, indiges-

tion, inflammation of the kidneys, inflammation of the pancreas, joint pain, depression, itching, hives, change in skin
color, hair loss, ingrown toenails with or without infection,
crystals in the urine and numbness of the mouth.

· Lopinavir/ritonavir (Kaletra) is a combination of Lopinavir
and ritonavir. The most commonly reported side effects are
abdominal pain, abnormal bowel movements, diarrhea,
feeling weak and/or tired, headache and nausea.

Children taking Kaletra may sometimes get a skin rash.
Liver problems, sometimes severe, may occur in patients,
as may pancreatitis, which may also be severe. Some
patients have large increases in triglycerides and cholesterol. Diabetes and high blood sugar may occur in patients
taking protease inhibitors such as Kaletra. Changes in body
fat have also been seen in some patients taking antiretroviral therapy. And some patients with hemophilia have
increased bleeding with protease inhibitors.

· Nelfinavir mesylate (Viracept). The most common side
effect is diarrhea. Other side effects include nausea, gas
and rash. Diabetes and high blood sugar (hyperglycemia)
may also occur. Changes in body fat in patients taking antiretroviral therapy may occur. Some patients with hemophilia may have increased bleeding with protease
inhibitors.

· Ritonavir(Norvir). Side effects include feeling week/tired,
nausea, vomiting, loss of appetite, abdominal pain,

changes in taste, numbness and tingling of the hands or feet or around the lips, headache and dizziness. Liver problems, sometimes severe, may occur in patients, as may pancreatitis, which may also be severe. Some patients have large increases in triglycerides and cholesterol. Diabetes and high blood sugar may also occur. Allergic reactions can range from mild to severe. Some patients with hemophilia may have increased bleeding with protease inhibitors. Some patients taking anti-HIV medicines may also have changes in body fat.

· Saquinavir (Invirase) (hard gel form), or Fortovase (soft gel) may cause diarrhea, nausea, abdominal discomfort and heartburn. Other side effects include abdominal pain, gas, vomiting, fatigue, headache, body aches, anxiety, depression, warts, change in sexual appetite, taste changes, constipation, sleeplessness, weight gain, gum disease, numbness or tingling, fever, convulsions, itching and rash, shortness of breath, fungal infection, hepatitis, night sweats, blurred vision, difficult urination, dizziness, coughing blood, bleeding in the brain, ulcers, inflamed pancreas and rapid heart rate. Increases in liver function tests, diabetes increased blood sugar levels and have been reported; changes in body fat have also been reported.

### *Fusion Inhibitors*

Fusion inhibitors, one of the newest treatments for HIV, prevent the attachment of the virus to the CD4 receptor on the cell surface. In short, they block HIV's ability to infect healthy CD4 cells. They are to be used only with other anti-HIV medicines.

· Enfuvirtide (Fuzeon). Because enfuvirtide is injected, it can cause injection-site reactions, including itching, swelling, redness, pain or tenderness, hardened skin and bumps. Other side effects may include bacterial pneumonia, serious allergic reactions such as trouble breathing, fever with vomiting, skin rash, blood in the urine and swelling of the feet. Call your health care provider immediately if these reactions occur. Still other side effects, in combination with other anti-HIV medicines, may include pain and numbness in feet or legs, loss of sleep, depression, weakness or loss of strength, muscle pain, decreased appetite, constipation and pancreas problems.

## TREATMENT OF SIDE EFFECTS

### Diarrhea

Call your health care provider if you have diarrhea that lasts for more than two days. It is important to make sure that an intestinal infection or parasite is not causing the diarrhea. If you have a temperature, or if the diarrhea has mucus or blood mixed with it, it is more likely the diarrhea is from an infectious cause. A stool specimen will help determine the cause.

The biggest danger with diarrhea is dehydration and loss of potassium. This can happen very quickly. You should note the frequency and volume you are putting out and try to replace it with a fluid that has electrolytes in it, such as broth, tea, bouillon, ginger ale, diluted orange juice. (Apple juice and dairy products often upset the stomach and increase the diarrhea.)

High fiber foods like fruit, vegetables and whole grain breads should be avoided during the diarrhea. Try plain rice, cream of wheat, white crackers with salt, white toast, and plain noodles with a small amount of butter.

The best way to treat diarrhea is to drink plenty of fluids and stop putting solid food into your stomach. Sometimes this is hard to do with a pill regimen that requires you to eat. Talk to your provider to work out a plan. Don't wait until you are dehydrated to get help.

### Nausea

Many antiretrovirals can cause nausea and vomiting. The vomiting usually occurs less than five times per day and in relatively small volumes. These symptoms subside as your body adjusts to the drug. If you have nausea for more than a week, to the point where it is interfering with your ability to eat, call your provider. It could indicate another problem, and if it is severe it should be evaluated. If you are vomiting for more than two days, or are having trouble keeping up with the fluid losses (can't keep replacement fluids down), call your provider. The provider may want to check you to make sure you do not have a serious problem such as a gastrointestinal infection or food poisoning.

## LONG-TERM SIDE EFFECTS

Thinning of the arms and putting fat on the trunk is a phenomenon seen in people on antiretrovirals for long periods of time (years). This side effect is rare, but it has received a lot of attention lately so I thought we should explain it. Basically, people gain weight around their middle but lose weight in their arms and legs. If you have been on ARVs and are putting on inches around your waist and your arms seem to be thinner, call your health care provider. It may be necessary to make a drug change.

Lipid abnormalities have been mentioned with each drug description, but they are mainly seen with protease inhibitors. Elevations of cholesterol and triglycerides are associated with an increased risk of coronary artery disease (heart attacks). Exercise and diet changes may help. If they do not, you should be treated with lipid-lowering drugs.

Diabetes mellitus (also known as hyperglycemia and elevated blood sugar) is associated with protease inhibitor use. It is seen more commonly in people who have a family history of diabetes or are overweight. It too needs to be treated with oral

---

*The best way to treat diarrhea is to drink plenty of fluids and stop putting solid food into your stomach. Sometimes this is hard to do with a pill regimen that requires you to eat. Talk to your health care provider to work out a plan. Don't wait until you are dehydrated to get help.*

---

hyperglycemics and, rarely, insulin, if dietary changes do not control it.

Lactic acidosis is thought to result from direct toxicity to the part of the cell called the "mitochondrion." This condition results in severe illness and requires emergency treatment and hospitalization. Suspected drugs are to be discontinued.

The symptoms of lactic acidosis are profound fatigue, malaise, and an increased rate of breathing, and it progresses rapidly. This condition requires an immediate evaluation in an emergency room.

## OTHER TREATMENTS

Drugs that increase your immune function, called "immunopotentiators," may also be part of your therapy. These drugs increase the CD4 count but should only be given when you are taking antiretrovirals and are fully suppressing viral replications.

# CHAPTER 7

# OPPORTUNISTIC INFECTIONS

If you have HIV, you may contract an opportunistic infection (OI) at some point, especially if your CD4 count drops below 200. By definition, opportunistic infections hit people with weakened immune systems. They usually crop up only when someone's CD4 becomes low, despite medications, or when someone with HIV has not been receiving regular medical care and has not been taking medicines to prevent the infection from taking hold.

In the 1980s and early '90s, people with HIV commonly died of opportunistic infections. But today, these infections have become less common among people with HIV who are receiving treatment. The antiretroviral medications restore immune function, keeping people strong enough to fight these infections. Also, even in the event that someone's CD4 count does become dangerously low, health care providers are very practiced in preventing and treating the infections. Drugs may be given to prevent an infection (a practice called "prophy-laxis"), or to treat the infection.

Sadly, the rates of opportunistic infections and their complications, including death, are higher among Black men and Black women. This isn't because Black Americans are more prone to the infections. It is largely because Black people do not receive medical care early enough. Black people tend not to call a health care provider when they feel sick—even long after symptoms have been present. This practice of not getting medical help, a practice all too common in our community, results in people getting diagnosed later and getting care at late stages of a disease, be it HIV, cancer, diabetes or heart disease.

*In the 1980s and early '90s, people with HIV commonly died of opportunistic infections. But today, these infections have become less common among people with HIV who are receiving treatment.*

That's true even of people who were diagnosed years earlier and knew they were HIV positive. As a result, they die sooner. Even if you are mistrustful of the medical establishment and just don't feel comfortable in a doctor's office, or if, in the past, you didn't keep your appointments, you can change because your life depends on it. You need to take responsibility for your health and take control of your life. You're already dong this by learning about your disease, so that you can communicate better with your health care provider and start anticipating problems before they occur. Now your life depends on your helping to establish a good working relationship with your provider.

*Make the medical system your own.* The health care providers who treat HIV patients consider it a 24-hour job. Once you contact them, they'll give you a phone number to reach them or their associates at any time. Call if you find yourself feeling ill. The threat of opportunistic infection is real, especially if your CD4 count is less than 200. This threat is another good reason to get the medical care that you deserve and that is there for you. *Other patients have learned to be proactive about their health. You can, too.*

Opportunistic infections are diseases that a healthy person easily fights off. Someone with a damaged immune system, such as people with HIV or on chemotherapy for cancer, have little natural defense against them. Opportunistic infections are caused by bacteria, fungi, parasites and viruses normally found all around us. They make people with HIV sick because people with HIV do not have the immunity to fight them. Some of these infections such as thrush, a yeast infection of the mouth and throat, are merely a nuisance. Others, such as PCP, a type of pneumonia, are deadly if they go untreated.

Getting an opportunistic infection is a sign that your immune system is unable to fight off the infection. If you develop an opportunistic infection and/or your CD4 cell

---

*If you develop an opportunistic infection and/or your CD4 cell count drops to 200 or less, your HIV has progressed to AIDS. The infection must be treated and you have to do your best to increase your CD4 count by taking antiretroviral drugs and taking good care of yourself.*

---

count drops to 200 or less, your HIV has progressed to AIDS. The infection must be treated and you have to do your best to increase your CD4 count by taking antiretroviral drugs and taking good care of yourself. As your CD4 count increases above 200, there is less chance that you will get an opportunistic infection.

During your first visits, the health care provider may test you to see if you have been exposed to any of the common opportunistic infections. Some of the tests may come back positive. Don't be alarmed! Some tests merely show if you have been exposed to the germ in the past, not that you are sick with the infection. Depending on the germ and the strength of your immune system, you may or may not be treated.

*Some tests merely show if you have been exposed to the germ in the past, not that you are sick with the infection.*

In the 1980s, before it was commonplace to use such drugs, many people with HIV contracted PCP and died from it. Other people developed dangerous infections of the blood and liver. Today, in the United States and other "developed" countries, these diseases are far less common. These diseases are common abroad in poor countries where medical care and drugs are inadequate. But for most Americans, at least, antiretroviral drugs have completely changed the natural history of HIV and have thereby changed the outlook for people with HIV and AIDS.

*If your CD4 dips below 200 you become more vulnerable to opportunistic infections. Even if you are having no symptoms, your provider probably will prescribe antibiotics or other drugs to prevent you from getting ill.* Even though some of the newly prescribed drugs may have side effects, research shows that it is worth it for HIV patients to take these drugs. The benefits far outweigh the risks.

Here are some of the more common opportunistic infections. If you notice any of these symptoms in yourself or someone you know who has HIV, see your provider immediately!

---

# COMMON OPPORTUNISTIC INFECTIONS

*Cytomegalovirus,* (CMV), can be an eye, gastrointestinal, lung, and nervous system virus. It occurs at CD4 counts below 50. When CMV causes eye disease, it can cause blindness, but if it is caught early enough it can be treated. CMV is best detected by a special exam conducted by an eye doctor (an ophthalmologist). An early exam gives the eye doctor the opportunity to spot the disease before your vision is harmed. You should have this exam when your CD4 count is 100 or less. You must immediately report any changes in your eyesight to your provider.

*Kaposi's sarcoma* is a skin cancer. Kaposi's causes a purple raised area in light-skinned people and a brown area in those with darker complexions. It may be on your face, lower legs or feet, genital area, or chest. In your mouth, Kaposi's usually shows up as a red, raised area on the roof of your mouth. It

may also be found on your gums, tongue or tonsils. It is now
known to be associated with herpes virus 8 infections. This
organism often infects the lining cells of veins and arteries,
causing them to develop the cancerous growth.

*Mycobacterium avium complex,* or MAC. Occurs at CD4
counts under 50. It is caused by an organism found widely in
the environment. In humans, it causes pneumonia and an
infection centered in the GI tract blood. Symptoms to watch
for are high fever, stomach ache, diarrhea, serious weight loss
and profound fatigue. It is treated with an antibiotic or combination of antibiotics until the symptoms go away. You may
also take an antiobotic to prevent MAC infections.

*Pneumocystis carinii pneumonia,* or PCP. This lung infection
is caused by an organism that is now thought to be most
closely related to a fungus and not a protozoa. It is most
common at CD4 counts of 200 or less if someone is not
taking Septra@ or Bactrim@ (trimethoprim/sulfamethoxa-
zole) prophylaxis. Its symptoms start with low-grade fever,
shortness of breath upon exertion, and a non-productive
cough. These symptoms increase over one to three days to
profound shortness of breath at rest, together with a fever
and fatigue. PCP is a life-threatening illness and requires an
immediate visit to the emergency room or clinic. It is treated
and prevented with antibiotics. If you recognize these symptoms in someone who may have HIV, take him or her to the
emergency room immediately.

*Toxoplasmosis* or *toxo*. It occurs at CD4 counts under 100.
Toxo is caused by a single-celled organism called a protozoa. It
lives in a dormant state in the soil, in cat feces, and sometimes on fresh fruit and vegetables, and it is harmless to people who are healthy. But when it strikes people with HIV, it can
cause a serious brain infection. The symptoms of "toxo" may
be mild-to-moderate confusion, and personality changes.
Patients may complain of weakness of the face, hand or foot.
It is treated with a combination of drugs, which are taken for
life. To help prevent its recurrence:

·   Wear gloves and a mask when cleaning a cat litter box or
    get someone to do it for you.
·   Wear gloves when gardening.
·   Wash fresh fruits and vegetables before eating.

The drugs work by preventing the parasite from using a B vitamin, which we also need. So when people are treated for
toxo, they are also are given a B vitamin supplement.

*Tuberculosis (TB)* occurs at any CD4 level. TB is caused by a
mycobacterium and it usually infects the lungs, causing coughing, fever, sweats and, eventually, coughing up blood. You catch
TB from an infected person who is coughing or sneezing. TB is
easily caught in prison, shelters and any place where people
are in close contact. *Anyone with HIV who tests positive for
being exposed to TB is treated for it.* It can infect other organs,
too. TB is curable but it takes time. The drugs can kill the
organism only when it divides. It divides slowly, so the treat-

ment is long. Active TB is treated by taking four different antimycobacterial agents for two to three months, then three antibiotics for nine to twelve more months. Inactive TB, meaning that the patient tests positive but has no active disease (as defined by a clear chest X ray and negative sputum for TB), is treated with one drug, Isoniazide (INH), for up to one year.

*Candidiasis,* or *thrush*, occurs at any CD4 count as well as during the primary syndrome. Thrush, or candidasis in the mouth, is not officially described by the U.S. Centers for Disease Control (USCDC) as an opportunistic infection, though recurrent vaginal yeast infections are. Still, *thrush in adults is rarely seen in people with strong, healthy immune systems. It is often the first sign people have that they are infected with HIV.*

Thrush is caused by an overgrowth of yeast, a tiny organism that is present in everyone's mouth. Usually, it is kept in check by your immune system. With HIV, the yeast overgrows. It shows up as small, white spots on your tongue and inside of your mouth. The spots look like cottage cheese and they cause irritation. You may have a sore throat and the disease can spread to your esophagus and become very serious. Esophagus involvement requires treatment with strong antifungal medications. If you—or someone you know—have had oral thrush and haven't been tested for HIV, you or your friend need to get tested. Thrush can show up within weeks after a person has been exposed to HIV. (See "Primary HIV Syndrome" in Chapter 1.)

Vaginal yeast infections, another form of thrush, are very common. But if you or a friend have had more than five in one year, you should be tested for HIV. A vaginal yeast infection causes itching and burning in the vaginal area, with a white discharge that looks like cottage cheese. It is treated with creams inserted into the vagina or with drugs taken by mouth.

Candida esophagitis is a severe infection of the esophagus, the tube that connects your mouth with your stomach. It is characterized by difficulty swallowing or by pain on swallowing. Patients usually can point to the exact place the food "gets stuck" or causes pain. With instruments, providers can identify an area of candida growth in the wall of the esophagus. Treatment may require hospitalization, but in most cases patients can be treated on an outpatient basis with strong oral antifungal medications.

*Cryptococcal meningitis* usually occurs at CD4 counts of 100 and below. It is commonly found in dirt and is caused by a fungus that, once in the body, travels to the spine. This condition causes a fever and "the worst headache you have ever had in your life," followed by nausea and vomiting. It is known for being rapid in its onset, over a period of a few hours. This is an extremely dangerous disease and you must get to a hospital immediately for treatment. Diagnosis and treatment is serious and involves tapping the spine and removing some of the fluid, which is causing pressure in the brain. You will be given an intravenous drug (Amphotericin B) followed by an oral drug (Diflucan) to prevent recurrence of this condition.

Below is a description of other infections that commonly occur in people with HIV. Under the strict definitions of the U.S. Centers for Disease Control, they are not considered opportunistic infections.

# OTHER COMMON INFECTIONS

*Herpes Zoster (shingles)* occurs at any CD4 count. Shingles is a reactivation of a chicken pox infection you had when you were a child. The virus remains dormant in your nerve roots and, with a weakening of your immune system, breaks out. Shingles can be very painful. It can be treated with drugs.

*Skin infections* are very common with HIV, and become more of a problem at CD4 counts of 200 or less. They are usually caused by staphylococcus ("staf") or by strep infections, and can be treated with a topical antibiotic or oral antibiotic.

*Skin fungi,* including infections of the nails, cause the nail to turn yellow and weaken, then to turn black and fall off. Skin fungi can occur at any CD4 count, as the result of fungal infection of the nail beds. Antifungal creams or pills usually clear this infection up nicely, but it requires treatments that require months of therapy.

*Cat scratch disease* or *bacillary angiomatosis* can occur at any CD4 count. After a person is scratched by a cat, infection starts and causes lymph drainage in that area. This condition causes severe blistering of the skin along the distribution of the vein. It is easily treated with erythromycin-based antibiotics.

*Molluscum contagiosum* is a viral infection that looks like tiny, raised white, pearly bumps on the face or trunk, especially in shaving areas. It occurs at CD4 counts of 100 or less and often goes away with antiretroviral therapy. It is usually self-limited and does not require direct treatment. Treating the HIV with ARVs is the best course of action.

*Oral hairy leukoplakia* affects the side of the tongue and usually occurs at CD4 counts of 100 or less. Its symptoms are a white-grayish plaque on the tongue that looks like fish gills and can't be wiped off. This has been associated with a virus called Epstein-Barr. Treating the HIV with ARVs is the best course of action.

Remember, these infections are far more rare than they were ten years ago, and in most cases, if they are detected early, can be effectively treated.

# CHAPTER 8

# AIDS

Because health care providers and patients have learned so much in recent years about good care, the development of AIDS in those who have HIV is becoming less common. But it still happens. Strictly defined, AIDS means a CD4 count of 200 or less or an opportunistic infection in an HIV-positive patient. If this happens to you, don't panic. Don't give up hope. With careful attention to your antiretroviral medications and other care, you should be able to pull out of it and get your immune system working again.

Your provider's first goal will be to get your CD4 count up to a point where you are not so vulnerable. This may require starting ARVs or, if you are on ARVs already, switching to a new combination of drugs. At the same time, drugs are available to prevent and treat a number of the opportunistic infections. So, even though your CD4 count is low, with care you can remain free of infections.

As we mention in Chapter 6, "Antiretroviral Medications," you can get further help from drugs like Interleukin,® which are in a class called "immunopotentiators." These drugs focus on supporting the immune system when it no longer works well. In combination with ARVs, Interleukin can increase your CD4 count considerably and restore immune function even in patients who are severely depleted. This therapy is not accepted as standard, but is in experimental trials.

If you keep your appointments regularly, you and your health care provider will usually have some warning that your CD4 count is dropping before it becomes dangerously low. Especially in the African American community, people often don't go to a clinic or ER and get tested for HIV until they are sick with AIDS. The test comes back positive and the blood work shows a CD4 count of 200 or less. Or, quite commonly, a person goes to an emergency room because of a nagging, dry cough and shortness of breath, and it is discovered that he or she has PCP and AIDS.

If this is you or a friend, don't worry. You still have a strong chance of regaining your strength and immune function if you take antiretroviral medications as prescribed and take very good care of yourself. Especially if you have never taken anti-retroviral drugs, the odds are good that, with treatment, your CD4 count will go up to a safer zone. If you can get your CD4 count above 200, you are much less likely to get an opportunistic infection.

It is rare today to see AIDS develop in White, middle class people with HIV. But AIDS is still happening to African Americans. This isn't because the drugs work less well for them, or because Black people get AIDS more easily. It is because not enough Black people use the medical care available to them. The providers are there, the clinics are there, and the money is there to pay for the medications.

We all know what happened at Tuskegee. But today there's much less reason for Blacks to fear the medical establishment. What keeps HIV patients from the treatment and support they need—besides the general uneasiness in the Black community about medical institutions—are community stigmas about having HIV, about being gay or bisexual or transgender and about being a drug user. As long as these stigmas remain and the community is afraid to talk about them, AIDS will continue to plague us.

Don't let labels get in the way of getting good medical care. Don't label yourself and be prevented by shame from seeking help. Take the first step and you will find people who love and support you, who will help you overcome any misplaced shame you may have about HIV. HIV is no different from any other serious disease, like cancer. If you or a loved one is sick, you deserve the very best treatment, just as you would if you had cancer.

## LIVING WITH AIDS

At a CD4 count of 200 or less, you are at great risk for opportunistic infections, like PCP and toxoplasmosis. Opportunistic infections afflict people whose immune systems are compromised. (For detailed descriptions of opportunistic infections, see Chapter 7.)

People with these CD4 levels used to experience rapid declines in their health, including severe weight loss and chronic diarrhea. Today, such problems are not common in people who are cared for by a health care provider. In other parts of the world, where the needed health care just doesn't exist, the old problems remain. But here in the United States, we see these problems in people who deny themselves treatment with antiretrovirals.

The medicines work, but you must work, too. You have to take good care of yourself at this time and watch your health closely. You also need to stay in close touch with your health care provider and know whom to call in case of an emergency.

In Chapter 4, we described how to set up a support team and why it's important for you to do so. If you haven't done so already, make arrangements now for your care in the event that your condition worsens or you become ill with an opportunistic infection. If family and friends are unable to support you, contact an AIDS advocacy organization or a local church with an AIDS ministry.

---

*If you haven't done so already, make arrangements now for your care in the event that your condition worsens or you become ill with an opportunistic infection. If family and friends are unable to support you, contact an AIDS advocacy organization or a local church with an AIDS ministry.*

---

## WHAT TO WATCH OUT FOR

You may feel more fatigued than usual. Certain symptoms are warning lights that tell you to see your provider right away. The following symptoms may be signals that you have an opportunistic infection or that the virus is advancing rapidly:

- A fever of 101 or higher for more then two days
- A cough, dry or with phlegm, that lasts more than two days
- Shortness of breath with exertion
- A headache that gets worse over hours and feels like the worst headache of your life— especially if associated with a fever
- Weakness of face, hand or foot
- Change in your vision, loss of vision, double vision
- Persistent diarrhea, nausea or vomiting—especially with visible blood

## PREVENTING INFECTIONS

With a CD4 level of 200 or less, you are vulnerable to all types of infections. It makes sense now to wash your hands after being in public, to help prevent colds and flus. You must also:

- Avoid handling cat litter and raw meat or fish to reduce the possibility of contracting parasites
- Wear gloves when you expose yourself to dirt, as in gardening

- Be extra careful to drink bottled water if you go camping or travel to a foreign country
- Wear clean clothes to help prevent skin infections
- Bathe regularly

*With a CD4 count of 200 or less, you are vulnerable to all types of infections. It makes sense to wash your hands after being in public, to help prevent colds and flus.*

You may have more frequent and severe outbreaks of oral or genital herpes, fungal infections, skin infections, and thrush or vaginal yeast infections. Neither herpes nor yeast infections are life-threatening, but they can be uncomfortable. Both are treatable. (For more information about these infections, see Chapter 7.)

To help prevent you from getting certain opportunistic infections, including PCP, toxoplasmosis, bacterial pneumonia and mycobacterium avium complex( MAC), your provider may give you antibiotics to take each day (see Chapter 7).

## IMMUNE RECONSTITUTION

If you already have an opportunistic infection and are being treated for HIV with antiretrovirals for the first time, you may at first experience a worsening of those symptoms related to opportunistic infections. That is because until now your immune system has been too sick to fight the infections, but when it revs up after you start taking antiretrovirals, your immune system is able to send white cells into the infected areas, resulting in new symptoms.

While you are under antiretroviral treatment at a CD4 level of 50 or lower, you'll feel weak, especially in your ability to sustain physical activity, and you may need help with daily tasks such as cooking, cleaning and doing laundry. Anticipate the need for more rest, schedule frequent naps. They can be short, 30–90 minutes. If you need to stop and rest while you're in the middle of a task, do so. Rest is just fine.

Remember, even with a CD4 count of 0, you are still capable of becoming stronger, with the help of antiretroviral therapy. In many late-stage patients, especially in those who have never used antiretrovirals before, treatment brings the viral load down to undetectable levels and the CD4 counts increase. Even in patients with little response in viral load and CD4 count, disease progresses more slowly while they are taking ARVs.

## CHAPTER 9

# AFRICAN AMERICAN WOMEN AND HIV

HIV among women is growing and the rates are highest among Black American women. Jeanne Amber, in her article "Why Don't You Use a Condom?" (*Essence*, August 2002), reminds us that one in 3000 White women, one in 400 Latinas, and one in 160 Black women test positive for HIV. The leading causes of these high rates among Black women are 1) getting infected by men (40%), and 2) infection through drug use and unsterilized needles (27%.) In the United States, AIDS is the fourth leading cause of death among Black women ages twenty-five to forty-four, and in thirteen American cities it is the number one cause of death among them.

In Chapter 11, we will discuss HIV/AIDS and addiction. In this chapter, our concern is with that big 40 percent of Black women who are infected by men. Women in long-term relationships want to trust their men, and therefore usually do not think of themselves at risk. But they are. Look at it this

---

*Even the most wonderful partner may have taken risks before he met you—sometimes, risks he doesn't remember. Because of the taboos against promiscuity, injected drug use and homosexuality, men are often ashamed to reveal to a woman that she's at risk.*

---

way: Even in a loving, long-term relationship you are actually sleeping with everyone your partner has ever slept with. That's why it's important that *you* take the initiative, by insisting that you both get tested.

Even the most wonderful partner may have taken risks before he met you—sometimes, risks he doesn't remember. Because of the taboos against promiscuity, injected drug use and homosexuality, men are often ashamed to reveal to a woman that she's at risk.

Back in the early days of HIV/AIDS activism, one of the powerful slogans was "Silence=Death." That's still true today. Silence is the reason rates are soaring among women in general and Black women in particular. Sadly, many Black women only find out they are positive after they become pregnant.

Yes, it can be tough putting questions to a man about his earlier sexual life. But you don't need the details. You just need a commitment from him to go with you to get tested, no questions asked, so you both know.

It's more than time for Black women to take the initiative as part of a community turning to safe sex. True, many women (like many men) have a hard time talking about HIV and safer sex. But you must learn to be strong. That's the only way to protect yourself, the child who may come, and even your partner, who could be infected and not know it.

## IF YOU ALREADY HAVE HIV AND AREN'T PREGNANT

While we still have a lot to learn about women and HIV/AIDS, experience so far tells us that the virus progresses in women who are not pregnant the same way that it progresses in men, and that women respond just as well to antiretrovirals as men. The only difference we've discovered so far is that women often have lower CD4 levels than men at the same stage of the disease. In other words, a woman who has HIV for ten years may have a lower average CD4 count than a man who has had HIV for the same length of time. You should be aware of this small difference when your health care provider tries to talk to you about starting ARVs.

You may find that, with HIV, your menstrual cycles become erratic, heavier or lighter, with mid-cycle bleeding. Also, certain drugs and drugs used to treat opportunistic infections may cause menstrual irregularities.

Talk to your health care provider if you experience any of the following:

- *Heavy bleeding that makes you weak or anemic,*
- *Constant bleeding*
- *Unexpected mid-cycle bleeding*

It may be possible to switch you to different drugs that don't cause these problems. In some cases, birth control pills are prescribed as a way to control heavy bleeding. So talk to your health care provider. There is no need to put up with uncomfortable and potentially harmful irregularities that are easily treatable.

You may experience more vaginal infections or herpes than you have in the past. These infections are not life-threatening but can be very uncomfortable, so tell your health care provider, who will treat you. Yeast infections are caused by an overgrowth of the yeast naturally found in the vagina. They can be treated with vaginal creams or a pill. If you are getting yeast infections often, you can take steps to prevent them. You can help prevent them by wearing clean, all-cotton underwear with loose-fitting pants or skirts.

Yeast infections can also occur in the mouth, throat, and esophagus, and such infections occur in women more than men. Oral thrush can be prevented or treated with a mouth rinse. Thrush in the esophagus requires oral medication, and sometimes IV antifungals.

Women with HIV also are more prone to outbreaks of genital warts and to cervical cancer. *Cervical cancer is a severe, life-threatening, disease, so it is very important for you to have a gynecological exam including a test called a" Pap smear," at least once a year.* The health care provider will brush a few cells from your cervix and send them to a lab to be checked for abnormalities. Human papilloma virus (HPV), which causes warts, must be monitored, because it is also implicated in cervical cancer.

## BIRTH CONTROL

If you have HIV, prevent your partners from catching it by making sure they wear latex condoms. Or you may want to use a female condom. Either way, using a latex condom protects you from catching any new HIV infections or venereal diseases.

You may want to use other forms of birth control, such as pills, along with latex condoms. Your provider will discuss this with you. Some of the HIV drugs may decrease the effectiveness of birth control pills and need to be adjusted accordingly.

## IF YOU HAVE HIV AND ARE PREGNANT

If you have HIV and become pregnant, the same options are available to you as to every American woman:

- You may have and keep your baby, and with treatments, greatly decrease the chance that the baby will have HIV. Treatment may include AZT, Nevirapine (Viramune®), or AZT + 3TC. If your CD4 count is below 350, you will receive treatment with combination therapy.
- You can have the baby and offer him or her for adoption.
- You may terminate your pregnancy.

These choices are difficult, but they are choices you must make. Listen to other people's advice, certainly. But you're the one who must make the decision. Even if you decide not to follow through with the pregnancy, you should let your health care provider know that you are pregnant. Your anti-HIV medications may have to be adjusted, and besides, your provider will want to know what you are going through.

If you choose to have the baby, you should know that your HIV virus can be passed to your baby, especially during birth or through your breast milk. But today, you can take ARVs that help you stay well and reduce the chances that your baby will get your HIV.

*If you choose to have the baby, you should know that your HIV virus can be passed to your baby, especially during birth or through your breast milk.*

Antiretroviral drugs are recommended for pregnant women when the CD4 count is 350 or below. You will likely be given a "drug cocktail" of three drugs, as we describe in Chapter 6. The effects of these drugs on babies are largely unknown, and most of the reliable data is based on animal studies. In the table that follows you'll find the technical data on the risks of birth defects or cancer in the child.

While there are some risks, most women and babies tolerate the cocktail without problems. Research is still going on, but, to date, experts believe it is to the advantage of both mother and fetus for the mother to take ARVs.

Talk this over with your health care provider as early as possible. Most likely, he or she will encourage you to go on ARVs.

The cocktail is usually begun after the first three months of pregnancy. As you get closer to the birth, your provider may change the mix of drugs or switch you to AZT alone. If you take antiretroviral medications for those six months of your pregnancy and during delivery, the risk that your baby will have HIV will drop to less than five percent.

**Table 23. Preclinical and Clinical Data Relevant to Use of Antiretrovirals in Pregnancy**

| Antiretroviral Drug | FDA Pregnancy Category* | Placental Passage [Newborn:Maternal Drug Ratio] | Long-Term Animal Carcinogenicity Studies | Rodent Teratogen |
|---|---|---|---|---|
| zidovudine† | C | Yes (human) [0.85] | Positive (rodent, vaginal tumors) | Positive (near lethal dose) |
| zalcitabine | C | Yes (rhesus) [0.30 – 0.50] | Positive (rodent, thymic lymphomas) | Positive (hydrocephalus at high dose) |
| didanosine | B | Yes (human) [0.5] | Negative (no tumors, lifetime rodent study) | Negative |
| stavudine | C | Yes (rhesus) [0.76] | Positive (rodent, liver and bladder tumors) | Negative (but sternal bone calcium decreases) |
| lamivudine | C | Yes (human) [~1.0] | Negative (no tumors, lifetime rodent study) | Negative |
| abacavir | C | Yes (rats) | Not completed | Positive (anasarca and skeletal malformations at 1000 mg/kg [35x human exposure] during organogenesis) |
| saquinavir | B | Unknown | Not completed | Negative |
| indinavir | C | Yes (rats) ("Significant" in rats, low in rabbits) | Not completed | Negative (but extra ribs in rats) |
| ritonavir | B | Yes (rats) [mid-term fetus, 1.15; late-term fetus, 0.15 – 0.64] | Positive (rodent, liver tumors) | Negative (but cryptorchidism in rats)‡ |
| nelfinavir | B | Unknown | Not completed | Negative |
| amprenavir | C | Unknown | Not completed | Positive (thymic elongation; incomplete ossification of bones; low body weight) |
| lopinavir/ ritonavir | C | Lopinavir – yes (rats) [0.08 at 6 hrs post-dose] | Lopinavir – not completed. Ritonavir – see above | Negative (but delayed skeletal ossification and increase in skeletal variations in rats at maternally toxic doses) |
| nevirapine | C | Yes (human) [~1.0] | Not completed | Negative |
| delavirdine | C | Yes (rats) [late-term fetus, blood, 0.15; late-term fetus, liver 0.04] | Positive (rodent, liver and bladder tumors) | Ventricular septal defect |
| efavirenz | C | Yes (cynomolgus monkeys, rats, rabbits) [~1.0] | Not completed | Anencephaly; anophthalmia; microphthalmia (cynomolgus monkeys) |

* FDA Pregnancy Categories are:

A – Adequate and well-controlled studies of pregnant women fail to demonstrate a risk to the fetus during the first trimester of pregnancy (and there is no evidence of risk during later trimesters);

B – Animal reproduction studies fail to demonstrate a risk to the fetus and adequate and well-controlled studies of pregnant women have not been conducted;

C – Safety in human pregnancy has not been determined, animal studies are either positive for fetal risk or have not been conducted, and the drug should not be used unless the potential benefit outweighs the potential risk to the fetus;

D – Positive evidence of human fetal risk based on adverse reaction data from investigational or marketing experiences, but the potential benefits from the use of the drug in pregnant women may be acceptable despite its potential risks;

X – Studies in animals or reports of adverse reactions have indicated that the risk associated with the use of the drug for pregnant women clearly outweighs any possible benefit.

† Despite certain animal data showing potential teratogenicity of ZDV when near-lethal doses are given to pregnant rodents, considerable human data are available to date indicating that the risk to the fetus, if any, is extremely small when given to the pregnant mother beyond 14 weeks gestation. Follow-up for up to 6 years of age for 734 infants born to HIV-infected women who had in utero exposure to ZDV has not demonstrated any tumor development (184). However, no data are available on longer follow-up for late effects.

‡ These effects seen only at maternally toxic doses.

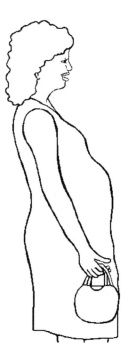

Even if you wait until the final months of your pregnancy, you can still be given drugs to decrease the chance of transmission. And even if you don't take the drugs until the delivery time, your baby's chance of getting your HIV can still be cut in half. Clearly, this is worth it.

Most women take advantage of these treatments, so that most babies born today to women with HIV are free of the disease. But of those babies who are born with HIV, almost all are Black American. What's going on? The drugs work just as well in Black women as in White.

The problem is that many Black women with HIV wait until close to the end of their pregnancies to get health care. Others *do* get to a provider earlier but don't take the treatments, or take them and then stop. Also, doctors and nurses in

ERs and delivery rooms need to make sure they offer IV AZT to women who present for the first time in labor. We can stop the terrible toll, protect our babies and invest in our common future simply by taking advantage of the treatments available to us.

Don't put your baby at risk. If you are pregnant, see your provider soon so that you, like other women in the U.S., can have the best treatment available. You and your baby deserve no less.

After birth, all babies will test positive for the virus because they have their mothers' antibodies. After six months, these antibodies will clear from the baby's blood and the babies will have their own antibodies.

> *Women with HIV should not breast-feed their infants. The newborn can contract HIV through breast milk, too. Use formula.*

The main risk of transmission from mother to baby is during labor. Taking AZT during gestation (after the first trimester), and during labor and delivery, as well as giving it to the baby orally at birth seems to be enough to prevent transmission.

During the first week after birth, you can find out if the virus is present in the baby's blood with a p-24 antigen or viral load test.

Women with HIV should *not* breast-feed their infants. The newborn can contract HIV through breast milk, too. Use formula. Research is being done in the developing world to look at continuing the HIV-negative baby on ARVs during breast feeding to prevent transmission. But in the United States, we recommend formula feeding alone.

We'd like you to take away some clear lessons from this chapter. As a woman and a potential mother, you owe it to yourself to do the following:

- Practice safe sex.
- Be sure to have yourself and your partner tested. Do it together.
- Report a pregnancy to your health care provider if you have HIV.
- Get the drugs you need to protect your baby from getting infected.
- Get the drugs you need to prevent your disease from progressing into AIDS.
- Don't breast-feed. Use formula.

# CHAPTER 10

# BEING BLACK AND GAY

## SILENCE=DEATH

Social stigmas against homosexual and bisexual behavior keep such behavior undercover. How such stigma works to spread HIV is obvious. Men who have had homosexual encounters but do not consider themselves to be homosexual are ashamed to reveal their history. Too often, women are reluctant to protect themselves when having sexual contact because they fear rejection. They believe they are in a monogamous relationship with a heterosexual men and do not perceive themselves to be at high risk for HIV. So they forget that each time they have sex they are having sex with all that man's previous partners.

> *Social stigmas against homosexual and bisexual behavior keep such behavior undercover.*

For all the commercialization of sex in this country, sex can still be a taboo subject, especially when it comes to being gay or bisexual, especially in the African American community. For some people, these subjects are wrapped in religion and morality, and they think gay sex a sin. For gay people, such taboos make it harder to reveal their homosexuality to their families or communities. The fact is that such fear often has no real base. Far more often, families offers love and support, whatever they may think about homosexuality in the abstract. Love can be more powerful than prejudice.

In fact, homosexuality has been with us since the beginning of time, and a number of cultures have lived comfortably with it, recognizing it as simply one of the many forms of human sexuality, and recognizing that individuals don't choose their sexuality: they simply *are* that way, whatever way that might be.

Now it's time for us to do what other cultures have done. We've made *some* beginnings. By law, if not always in practice, gays have won civil rights and protections from hate crimes. Too, in many parts of the country, people *are* talking openly about issues surrounding gayness, and some states now allow same sex marriages. But, sadly, there are still many communities, and regions of the country where discussion of gayness is still taboo.

There's no way to stop that deadly formula by which silence helps spread disease except by ending the veil of secrecy. Only when, as individuals and as a community, we can talk freely about our sexuality can we seriously begin to fight the HIV epidemic. When people are obliged to conduct their sexual lives underground, they're more likely to be involved in high-risk behaviors that lead to infection.

So the first part of the job belongs to the individual, along with his or her family and community. For the individual, the task is to be honest with yourself. Honesty leads to self-acceptance. Accepting yourself means loving yourself. You must love yourself first before you can truly love others.

The family's job is to accept the individual for who he or she is and not for what the family, or some family member, would like him or her to be. This is a hard lesson because it involves ideas of right and wrong, along with fear for the individual's well-being. In such cases, parents may feel they must "draw a line" on behavior they don't approve of. But drawing that line is exactly what parents need *not* do. The alternative that leads to a favorable outcome is for the parents and family to look into themselves, and to seek the reasons they feel as they do about their son's or daughter's sexuality.

If parents and family are honest with themselves, after a while they will recognize what is true: it is not a conscious choice that makes one homosexual, but something that comes from within. Once they see that, family members will also see that they needn't judge their son or daughter for a particular form of sexual expression. Instead, it is their job to love them unconditionally in their pursuit of their humanity.

The community's job is to understand the impact "community opinion" has on behaviors, especially sexual behavior. That impact can be positive or negative. Communities become positive forces, when community centers, including churches, become forums where people—*all* people—can freely speak their minds, and openly express to the community their fears and their needs. Already, many churches are extending their ministries to address the issues that surround HIV, and that surround gayness. In this way they are becoming a significant resource in the effort to stop the epidemic.

## THE CHURCHES AND THE EPIDEMIC

Some church leaders see the struggle to control the HIV epidemic as today's version of the civil rights movement. After all, the present threat against the community is great, as we know from the statistics. The Reverend Ronald Jeffrey Weatherford and Carole Boston Weatherford have written a book that views the struggle against the epidemic as another chapter of "the history of activism in the black church" *(Somebody's Knocking at Your Door,* Binghamton, N.Y.: The Haworth Pastoral Press, 1999).

Genevieve E. Bell has written a moving and practical memoir of her own struggle not to let her homosexual son's AIDS keep her from the refuge of the church. Her book, called *My Rose* (Cleveland, Ohio: Pilgrim Press, 1997), provides excellent study questions to help a ministry open discussions of HIV/AIDS and sexuality.

Prominent national voices are also being heard. Former Surgeon General Dr. David Satcher has spoken on how "unjust perceptions and stereotypes about gay men, injection drug users, their partners, and people living with AIDS" can keep them from seeking out testing and treatment that's available to them. He has urged the entire community, including the churches, to begin the discussion that can end these stereotypes and stigmas and to encourage people to seek out testing and the treatment that's available to them.

Helene Gayle, M.D., MPH, in her work as Director of the Center for HIV/AIDS, STDs and TB at the U.S. Centers for Disease Control and Prevention, has focused her center's resources on nurturing the development of community-based organizations, including churches, that can work closely with high-risk groups in the African American community. Dr. Gayle's initiative has made the Federal Government more effective in its own fight against the epidemic.

The Reverend Edwin C. Sanders, II, Pastor of the Metropolitan Interdenominational Church in Nashville, and Reverend Yvette Flunder, Senior Pastor and Founder of the United Church of Christ in San Francisco, both have dedicated large portions of their ministries to embrace and support people who are infected with HIV.

Organizations exist to help the churches become better able to help gay Black men and women and to help turn back the tide of HIV/AIDS. A group called Balm in Gilead (http://www.balmingilead.org), led by Pernessa C. Seele, encourages churches to start HIV/AIDS ministries and tells them how to do it. Balm in Gilead provides information about HIV/AIDS and what churches can do to help prevent it. This group is especially good at advising churches how to make their congregations more welcoming to people with HIV, through support services, understanding and love. For example, it shows how your church can provide a safe space so that members who are HIV-positive can reveal their disease to family and friends.

Useful, practical guides are also available. *Congregational Health: How to Make Your Congregation a Health-Aware Community*, by Kris Mauk, et al. (Roscoe, Illinois: Hilton Publishing, 2002) is a resource for health fellowships in ministries of all denominations.

## HONESTY AND SELF-ACCEPTANCE

But much work remains to be done. Some of it must begin with individuals, who are ready for openness and the healing that comes with it. This means being honest with yourself. If through unprotected sex or shared needles you have put yourself in danger of infection, get tested and, if appropriate, get treated. Let others whom you might infect know your history and your status, and use safe sex. Even if you don't choose to disclose your history and sexual preference, be honest in your *behavior* by practicing safe sex and not sharing needles.

At the core of all this is a simple human truth: human beings can't be whole until they accept all parts of themselves. Too many gay men and women, for too long, have felt obliged by prejudice and name-calling to conceal their identities from others, and to condemn themselves for being gay. The upshot is that, by internalizing the prejudices of others, they have been driven to lead secret closeted lives, and, too often, spread infection out of fear of being known.

Human sexual expression has many forms. Homosexuality and bisexuality are common and normal functions. By knowing this, the gay person finds self-acceptance, and the straight person stops being part of the problem. Once we can speak with each other on a common ground, human beings can give up the prejudices that make other human beings lead hidden lives.

## BEING TRANSGENDERED

The rates of HIV infections among transvestites in general are very high. Among male to female transgenders, the rate of infection is 35%. Rates among African Americans in this group, according to a recent article in the *Journal of Public Health,* are far higher—63%. This area is so hidden that we have barely done the basic research needed to understand the extent to which HIV has established itself in this special community.

Being transgendered means living with a heavy weight of stress and loneliness. If you are like many male-to-female transgendered people, you may have been pushed out, or fell out of, the mainstream workforce. You may have little money and no health insurance. You may work in the sex trade—a terribly dangerous activity. You may share the injection equipment that you use to administer hormones. Couple this behavior with HIV and you have another conduit by which the virus is entering the community.

The fact that you don't feel connected to either the gay community or the straight community means it is easy for you to feel isolated. That's exactly why you must create a safe and supportive community for yourself. You don't have to stay out in the cold. We all need human connection and human dialogue. That's what keeps us in this world. And for a person with HIV, feeling connected is doubly important. When you get isolated, it is hard to stay on track with your anti-HIV medications and the healthy lifestyle that will keep you well.

It is hard for you to develop a self-perception that is based on self-acceptance. Being African American has already put you in a "minority" posture with the dominant culture.

Homosexuals have learned how to be strong and function in the larger society in part by creating allegiances and associations with smaller aspects of society—professional groups, favorite sports teams, clubs, neighborhood, etc. But transgendered individuals are just beginning to see themselves as a group, and to create support systems focused on minimizing risk.

Every person deserves to feel like a human being and to be treated like one. But getting the treatment you need must start with self-help. You must seek out a counselor who can help you. Always keep in mind that you deserve the best for yourself, and that isolation and depression are bad for your spirit and your body that is fighting so hard for you against HIV.

> *Every person deserves to feel like a human being and to be treated like one.*

Counseling with a peer, or an understanding professional counselor, social worker, or pastor, can be the first step toward your new community. You'll learn to overcome the fear of misunderstanding that has kept you isolated and depressed, and, maybe, even stop blaming yourself for your sexual orientation and your HIV.

Get into medical care. Use your health care provider as a resource to help you find the support you need.

Regular meetings with a counselor can sustain your spirit and provide the discipline you need to keep yourself in the good health you deserve. The counselor can help you deal with the heavy pressures of your life, and in that way, help keep you emotionally on track. In addition, if you wish, your counselor can help you find your way out of the sex trade. Your counselor can do this by steering you toward other forms of employment, or finding social security or work disability benefits you may be entitled to, depending on the stage of your diagnosis. Your local AIDS advocacy organization also may be able to help you in these ways.

You can also help yourself. If you are a transgender who does sex work, wear condoms. If you are injecting hormones, don't share your equipment. Use clean needles. If you are sharing equipment, learn how to clean your works thoroughly with bleach (although this is not a foolproof way to avoid the virus and you're wiser not to share equipment). By using condoms and protecting yourself from contamination through shared needles, you protect yourself from contracting other strains of HIV. You also protect those you are involved with from catching your virus. *You can get free condoms at your local AIDS advocacy organization or AIDS clinic.*

Like everyone else infected with HIV, you, as a transgendered person, must help yourself by getting medicine and assistance for HIV, and by keeping regular appointments with your provider. If your life has been somewhat out of control, getting into these good habits will probably be hard at first. But soon you'll find that by taking care of yourself you renew your faith in yourself and in your ability to live a safe life as a transgendered person. Others have learned to do this and you can too.

If you do not have health insurance or money, your counselor, your AIDS advocacy group, and section 12 of the Resource section at the end of this book can help you find the assistance you need.

Many health care providers welcome transgendered patients. If at all possible, choose such a provider—someone you can comfortably talk to about your particualr health issues.

What's true for everyone is true for you: you must have people in your life who know you and understand your struggles. It doesn't matter whether you're looking into the eyes of a friend, a family member, someone in your support group, your provider, counselor, or social worker.

Support groups for transgendered people are still rare. The "movement" is young. But there *are* such groups, particularly in San Francisco, Boston and New York. Another way to connect with transgendered people is online. For a start, check out the web sites listed in section 12 of the Resource section.

# CHAPTER 11

# HIV/AIDS AND ADDICTION

If you are addicted to drugs or alcohol, you will be urged to go through detox and a substance abuse program. Half of all new cases of HIV are contracted through IV drug use. More than 57 percent of women with HIV caught it from IV drug use or from having sex with addicts or ex-addicts.

Remember: a sexual partner who was a drug addict ten years ago but is now clean may be harboring HIV, even if he or she doesn't have any symptoms yet. Only a test would show if the partner has HIV.

It's best for you to go through detox and begin the reha-bilitation process, which is lifelong. More than 70 percent of babies with HIV get the disease through a mother who was infected by an IV user or who uses herself.

Some inpatient detox wards work closely with HIV providers, so you may be able to begin therapy at the same

---

*It's best for you to go through detox and begin the rehabilitation process, which is lifelong. More than 70 percent of babies with HIV get the disease through a mother who was infected by an IV user or who uses herself.*

---

time as or shortly after detox. If you are addicted to drugs or alcohol, your health care provider will pay special attention to your health before you begin antiretrovirals. If you have been an IV drug user, you should be tested for Hepatitis B and Hepatitis C. You should discuss the indications for treating Hepatitis B and Hepatitis C, in the setting of HIV, with your provider. Your liver needs to be strong enough to handle the anti-HIV drugs. In addition, there are specific considerations that impact the choice of ARVS.

If you have been using heroin, you may be placed on methadone maintenance. Methadone mimics heroin without the heavy "high" feeling. You can function on it and think clearly. Most methadone programs require a daily visit for you to drink your methadone. The goal is to keep you off heroin. Giving high doses of methadone to people in maintenance assures the lowest relapse rates.

Some people take methadone for the rest of their lives and live normally. Others go through methadone tapering so that they will be completely free of drug addiction.

Many methadone clinics now include an HIV treatment on site, so you can be seen for your HIV when you receive your methadone. You can begin antiretroviral therapy while on methadone, but doses of certain antiretrovirals or your methadone may have to be adjusted upward.

There is no replacement drug like methadone to help addicts of other injectable drugs, such as cocaine or metamphetamine.

Once you have successfully completed detox, your job is to stay clean and allow your body to fight HIV with all its strength. Get the support you need to do this. And, above all, stay in the group. Keep your head clear and take responsibility for your actions. Practice safe sex by using a condom and not sharing IV equipment.

If you haven't gone through detox or you slip up and start using again, don't share needles and don't have sex without a condom. Keep detox in mind as your goal. Maybe you must wait until there is a space available for you. Hang in there, and keep in your mind's eye the new life that awaits you.

Alcoholics Anonymous and Narcotics Anonymous have proven very helpful for people recovering from alcohol or drug abuse.

If you are still using heroin, keep in mind:

- You can spread your virus or get someone else's from the needle or from droplets of blood on the paraphernalia (works).
- Never share equipment. It is best to use new equipment, but if you don't, clean yours after each use with cold water and full strength bleach rinses. The virus can live in a used needle for a number of weeks. Bleach doesn't necessarily protect you from getting HIV from

somebody else's works. Be sure to do a thorough job of cleaning, and use the bleach at full strength.

Your substance abuse group or counselor should have given you an emergency number to call if you start to feel bad, or if you want to get high again. Keep this number with you and use it! When those feelings come up, reach out. Work closely with your group and or/counselor. The more seriously you take that work, the less likely you are to experience these emergency situations.

## YOUR NEW LIFE

If you've decided to give up drugs and alcohol, you face big lifestyle changes—nearly all of them for the better. You're helping your body use *all* its resources to fight HIV. If your heart has been damaged by substance abuse, it too can recover, though this takes time. It took you years to get to where you are, so be willing to give some time to getting back to where you want to be. Try to be patient.

It's a little like someone unweaving a fabric in order to weave it again into a new design. You need to undo an entire lifestyle—the people you hang out with, your daily activities, and the activities and responsibilities you have avoided. If you put honest effort into this and get support, your chances of succeeding go way, way up. Even if you fail, try again. I know many patients who failed methadone maintenance or detox three times, only to succeed on attempt number four.

Being substance-free will give you a clearer picture of your life. You may have to work hard to regain the trust of those closest to you, who were pushed away by your behavior that was brought on by your addiction. To become more whole and be able to recover, you have to face up to the behaviors you were involved in while you were an abuser. You must admit to yourself and others that you weren't there for them, that you hurt them and that you are sorry. You can't lie to yourself or others about your behavior. It was damaging to everyone around you—but especially to yourself. Once you've honestly faced the people you've hurt, you can begin to heal them and yourself.

What has kept others in recovery and can inspire you is merely looking at two pictures: your life as a user as against the new life you can have. It is never too late. You may not be able to achieve the dreams you had before you were an addict. But now you can come up with new dreams, realistic ones that you

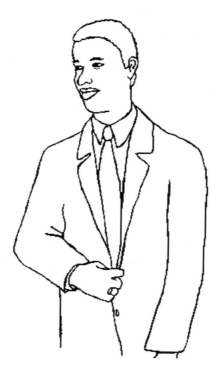

> *There is promise in each moment. Even in this instant, as you read, you can make a decision that will make all the difference in the world. The first step is yours. Be smart enough to define the support you need. That's a big step toward giving yourself a chance to put your life back in balance.*

*can* achieve—dreams that may lead you to a life based on honesty with yourself, which is the foundation of self-love and self-respect.

It is important to have dreams and to see the promise that today and tomorrow hold. There is promise in each moment. Even in this instant, as you read, you can make a decision that will make all the difference in the world. The first step is yours. Be smart enough to define the support you need. That's a big step toward giving yourself a chance to put your life back in balance.

# CHAPTER 12

# WELLNESS

Three good meals + exercise + good sleep = fewer complications of HIV. Stick to that simple formula and you'll not only get ill less often with complications of HIV, but you will also feel better and have more energy when you aren't ill.

You may not be used to eating well and taking good care of yourself. Many Americans live fast lives. We catch food on the run and rarely cook a full dinner for our families and ourselves. But fast food is generally bad food. High in fat and

---

*Three good meals + exercise + good sleep = fewer complications of HIV. Stick to that simple formula and you'll not only get ill less often with complications of HIV, but you will also feel better and have more energy when you aren't ill.*

---

calories and low in vitamins and fiber, fast food can do a number on your digestive system. Home-cooked, balanced meals, especially when they are lower in fat and high in fiber and life-giving vitamins and minerals, are superior.

*Home-cooked, balanced meals, especially when they are lower in fat and high in fiber and life-giving vitamins and minerals, are superior.*

Just as we African Americans rely too much on fast food, we tend to avoid exercise. Often, that means staying inside when it would do us more good to get out and around. It also means that we are likely to take a bus or drive when we could take a walk that would be beneficial to our health. Walking outdoors is nature's best exercise.

People with HIV who take care of themselves, give proper regard to their bodies, pay attention to what they eat and drink and get their heart pumping daily are likely to be strong and vital people. If they happen to be people with HIV, they are people who will feel sick far less often than people who don't exercise.

Getting a good sleep can be a problem. We bring the stress of the day to bed with us. Often, we've been revved up all day and find it hard to turn the volume down. Having HIV itself can obviously be an agitating experience that, if we don't do anything for stress management, can drive us to the edge. But some ways we use to manage stress cause more harm than help. Excessive alcohol or drugs are very bad medicine for people with HIV. Or we may just turn on the TV to relax, but what we get is designed to keep us in that revved-up state.

## A BRIGHT NEW LIFE

If you've been a drug or alcohol abuser, you may not have thought about your lifestyle in a long time. You've been too focused on your habit. But now you've been invited, and accept the invitation, to a new life. You accept it because you're a human being who wants to live as long as possible and to live the best you can. That means taking care of yourself, learning how to relax, giving your body what it needs (like healthy meals you cook for yourself) and exercise. It means getting rid of the activities that drain energy and weaken you.

As you go through detox and quit your habit, you'll begin to have the kind of experiences you may not have had in a long time. You'll learn to be kind to yourself, not in a selfish or greedy way, but as part of becoming that respectable, healthy adult you always wanted to be. Maybe you can remember how good you felt back when you *did* take care of yourself. Or maybe you can't. But that life and that good feeling are yours for the taking right now, at this very minute. You need only to reach out now for the help you need to make the necessary changes.

The first step is as plain as the nose on your face: See a counselor who can teach you how to reduce stress, help you get

---

*You may be surprised to find out that a diagnosis of HIV can be an opportunity for you to live better, to make it a priority to relax, to cook good meals for yourself, and to appreciate your body by giving yourself exercise and by getting rid of activities that hurt you.*

---

into detox and guide you back onto the path to better health. You may be surprised to find out that a diagnosis of HIV can be an opportunity for you to live better, to make it a priority to relax, to cook good meals for yourself, and to appreciate your body by giving yourself exercise and by getting rid of activities that hurt you.

As you begin making the necessary changes, you may have to distance yourself from your friends who aren't ready to make changes, and who continue to live self-destructively. Sure, that can be a bitter loss. These old friends are people you've come to depend on, even if they're not always dependable. But you'll find that as you make the changes you need in order to live well despite HIV, you will draw people to you who also live this way. So don't be afraid of being lonely for a while.

Your HIV or addiction support group can lend you a hand in making these changes. Lifestyle, eating well, taking vitamins and HIV medications—those are among the big topics at these meetings. If you haven't done so already, link up with an HIV support group now through your local AIDS advocacy organization.

Changes don't happen overnight. To make the changes you need, the changes we describe below, start small and be patient. You'll do best if you think of these changes as a gift to yourself first. Sure, those who love you will benefit, too. But it starts with you: be determined to give the gift of life to yourself.

## MAKING CHANGES

*The key to making these changes is to go slowly and take it step by step.* For example, if you have been advised to eat foods with

# Keep Your Household Infection-free

Keep in mind that while you're protecting your own health, you are also protecting the health of others. Yes, that means using condoms. But it also means taking ordinary precautions in a household where you're living with others. What it boils down to is this advice from the Centers for Disease Control about any setting, including the home, where such contact might occur:

· Gloves should be worn during contact with blood or other body fluids that could contain visible blood, such as urine, feces or vomit.

· Cuts, sores or breaks on both the care giver's and patient's exposed skin should be covered with bandages.

· Hands and other parts of the body should be washed immediately after contact with blood or other body fluids, and surfaces soiled with blood should be disinfected.

· Practices that increase the likelihood of blood contact, such as sharing of razors and toothbrushes, should not be done.

· Needles and other sharp instruments should be used only when medically necessary, and handled according to recommendations for health-care settings.

· Do not put caps back on needles by hand or remove needles from syringes.

· Dispose of needles in puncture proof containers out of reach of children and visitors.

potassium, like fresh fruit, don't expect to make yourself a fruit eater overnight. Sure, some people make changes like that. But for most of us slow and steady is the better way. Try eating one extra piece of fruit a day. Do this for a few weeks. Soon, it will feel normal, as if fruit has always been part of your regular diet. Before long, it will be easy to add more fruit, gradually, until you reach your target.

> *Before you begin making any changes in your lifestyle, find out from your provider or nutritionist exactly what you are to do.*

Before you begin making any changes in your lifestyle, find out from your health care provider or nutritionist exactly what you are to do. If it's a question of diet, find out what you are to eat and not to eat, the total calories you should take in each day, the amount of salt you are allowed. Other questions may come up aimed at your specific health condition.

If the change involves exercise, talk with the provider about what kind of exercise to do, for how long each time, how many times a week, and where to do it.

Working with your health care provider will feel good to you. You'll feel that you have a team behind you, people who want to do everything in their power to give you good health.

You will only begin to make a change when you are ready. Your level of readiness is the state of mind that determines how you make the many decisions that go into a particular kind of behavior. When you are stuck in a rut, you are in a low state of readiness to change.

You can also understand "level of readiness" from another point of view. The comedian Lenny Bruce used to say, "You gotta wanna." For you, now, the question is how badly do you "wanna"? You face this question every day, in ordinary things. You're lying around in your room, but you see the sun's shining and you think about taking a walk. How badly do you "wanna"?

If you're "not ready," maybe you never even thought about making life changes, or you did think about it, but couldn't see how the changing would do you any good. But maybe getting ready isn't as hard as it seems. You need to take a look at people who *are* ready, and people who have already made the changes—that is, people in your support group. These people have become confident about change because they've done the work, they've learned what they had to, one step at a time, one day at a time.

Or maybe they're like you, just now, for the first time, thinking through the problem and resolving to make the best of it. You're almost ready. You think about exercising, or diet, or keeping in closer touch with your support group, but you just can't seem to get started. Ask yourself right now, while you're reading these words: "Am I ready? Do I 'wanna'?" Depending on your answer, you and your counselor or support group can work out different approaches to moving you towards being ready, instead of staying stuck in the same old behaviors.

Be honest with yourself about what you can realistically achieve and how fast you can achieve it. But most urgently, be forgiving of yourself. Bad behavior in the past is in the past, water under the bridge. Now is the beginning of your future.

After you begin, on some days you'll experience resistance, a kind of negative voice inside that keeps whining: "Why don't I get to eat my favorite foods anymore?" and "Why am I getting up early every morning to take a walk?" Let that negative voice have its say. Just remind yourself of the strong truth you stand on: you're doing it because it will pay off. If you're watching what you eat, getting exercise, taking your meds, seeing your health care provider, staying in touch with your counselor and your support group, you're doing it because it pays off. You get sick less often and feel good more often. You look better and your mind's sharper. You feel a strong pride you may not have felt before, a pride in taking responsibility for your own life.

*Just remind yourself of the strong truth you stand on: you're doing it because it will pay off.*

You'll see long-range benefits as well. For some people, that may mean wanting to live long enough to see the grand-children grow up. Others just want to go on working at a job they love, or taking care of a child. Some people want to be a good example to their children. Others simply want not to depend on others to care for them, and that becomes their reason for taking care of themselves.

One last word about resistance, the voice that tells you you can't change. Everybody hears that voice. What can make that voice so strong is a person's lack of confidence, the feeling that "I don't have what it takes." Or maybe up to now you just didn't know where to start.

Whatever your reasons, when the subject of change comes up, you say things like "No matter how hard I try, I just can't seem to remember to take my pills." Or: "How can I eat the right things when my family still wants me to fix the foods I'm not supposed to eat?" Or: "I know a lot of people who started taking morning walks but only one who kept it up."

Lack of confidence is a hurdle that you can get over. You can build confidence by starting small—as in the example of adding fruit to your diet. Each small success will give you more confidence in your ability to succeed at even bigger tasks and to develop the will to get up and do it again, day after day.

It's as simple as that. Talk to somebody who exercises with weights. He or she will tell you the same thing. Maybe at the start you can barely handle a five-pound weight. Keep it up, and before long ten pounds will feel too light.

## Simple Changes to Reduce Your Risk of Infections

If your CD4 count is 200 or less, you will be more prone to infections of all kinds, ranging from colds and flus to skin infections and opportunistic infections. By making a few simple changes, you can help protect yourself.

*Safe Sex*

Having safe sex is one of the most important ways to take good care of yourself. For men, safe sex means wearing a condom when you have vaginal or anal sex, and during oral sex if you ejaculate, or come, in someone's mouth. It means that when you don't have a condom with you, you and your partner should use mutual stimulation instead. Many people find this unexpectedly sexy!

*Clean needles*

If you are still shooting drugs or hormones, find out from your provider where to get clean needles through your local needle exchange program. In many states syringes can be sold without a doctor's prescription. Remember, even if you are HIV-positive, the chance that you will contract another population of HIV when you use someone else's needle is very high. The chance that you will give your HIV to those who use a needle you have used is also very high.

*Cleanliness*

With HIV, you will be more prone to get skin infections and other infections. If you haven't paid much attention to wearing clean clothes, showering daily and having a clean living space, you should begin now if you want to reduce your chances of getting infections.

- Wash your clothes weekly and shower daily with mild soap. If you share your living quarters with other people you may want to start using your own washcloth and bar soap, or use liquid soap. Some infections (*not HIV*) can be spread by sharing a bar of soap.
- If you are weak and cannot get your clothes to the laundromat or clean your apartment, tell your AIDS advocacy organization or the AIDS mission at your church. Other people may be able to pitch in until you are back on your feet. Don't feel bad about asking. When you are well, you can volunteer to help others in the same way.

- When you clean your apartment, work in your garden, or clean a litter box, wear gloves and wash your hands afterwards. Germs live in soil but people with healthy immune systems fight off these diseases. People with compromised immune systems are vulnerable to a number of serious, even deadly, infections that are carried by germs in soil and cat feces. Wearing gloves will keep you from coming into contact with them.
- Wash your hands often. Washing hands cuts down on colds and flus. If you want to avoid getting colds and flus from people you know or the public, wash your hands at least six times a day, each time you come back home from running errands or being out with friends. Also, because there tends to be a lot of bacteria in the bathroom, keep your toothbrush in a cabinet in the bathroom or in another room.
- Don't share food and cigarettes. Other people have the ability to fight off colds and flus, but HIV may reduce your immunity. So while other people can share a forkful of food with someone who has a cold or a herpes infection and not get sick, you may not have that same protection. It's best not to share food or cigarettes with others.

## Food Safety

Eating is such a pleasurable experience that it may seem odd to associate foods with disease. But the truth is that many

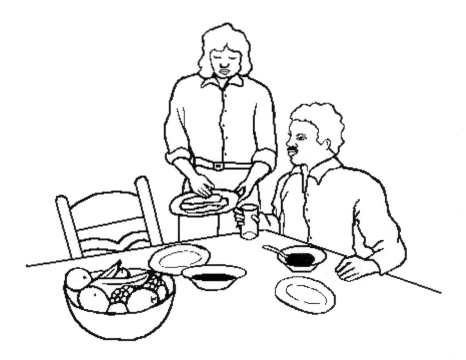

foods contain bacteria and other organisms, germs our normal immune systems knock out.

People with compromised immune systems need to be especially careful. Here are some suggestions for people with low CD4 counts (less than 200) as to how to avoid food-borne illnesses:

- Before preparing or eating your food, wash your hands thoroughly. Raw meat, chicken, fish and eggs can harbor harmful bacteria.
- Eat eggs that are thoroughly cooked (no over easy, sunny-side-up, or runny yolks). Avoid homemade mayonnaise and salad dressings that contain raw egg, and

eggnog and mousse, unless you know they were made in a sanitary manner and refrigerated.

- Eat only cooked fish and well-cooked meat.
- Eat foods that are pasteurized, including pasteurized cheeses, milk, cider and fruit juices.
- If you eat ice cream, make sure it is kept frozen solid in your freezer.
- Use a separate cutting board for meat and fish.
- Thoroughly wash your cutting board and knives in hot, soapy water every time you prepare meat or fish.
- Keep raw fish in the refrigerator for no more than twenty-four hours before cooking it—except shellfish, shrimp, lobster and crab, which must be eaten within hours after you buy it.
- Keep raw meat in the refrigerator for no longer than two days. Get in the habit of freezing meats you aren't going to use right away.
- If you keep leftovers of cooked meat, vegetables or grains, eat them within three days or throw them out. This precaution is very important for rice, which can grow bacteria called "listeria." Listeria can cause flu-like symptoms, followed by a type of encephalitis with fever and, in rare cases, paralysis.
- A good way to clean kitchen counters after handling raw meat or fish is to use a mixture of bleach: one teaspoon of bleach to a pint of water.
- Grungy sponges are bad. They can be run through the dishwasher or put in the microwave to help sterilize them.
- Rinse all fruits and vegetables before eating them.

- When you eat out, send back any food that does not appear to be thoroughly cooked or hot and send back any service-wear that is not clean.
- When ordering food, avoid raw salads and fruit, including salad bars, which harbor bacteria in foods that have been at room temperature for many hours.
- A word to the wise is to avoid soft serve ice cream. The machines may carry bacteria that can cause food poisoning.

## Quitting Smoking

You already know that smoking is bad for you and perhaps you have tried to quit. Now is the time. Some experts feel that if you are getting rid of drugs and/or alcohol at the same time, you should wait until you are through the detox before you quit smoking. But smoking is bad. It wears down the body in many ways. Smokers are more prone to colds and sinus infections, bronchitis and, of course, lung cancer. People with HIV who smoke increase their risk of emphysema, heart disease, and cancer significantly. Why play Russian roulette? Stop now.

Talk to your provider about nicotine gum or patches, or both. These have helped people through the acute nicotine withdrawal period, which normally lasts only one or two weeks. The psychological dependence is the harder habit to break, and often takes months.

The National Heart, Lung, and Blood Institute has worked out a useful list of ways to cope with withdrawal symptoms:

# COPING WITH WITHDRAWAL SYMPTOMS

| Withdrawal Symptom | Things You Might Do |
| --- | --- |
| Craving for Cigarettes | Do something else; take slow deep breaths; tell yourself, "Don't do it." |
| Anxiety | Take slow deep breaths; don't drink caffeine drinks; do other things. |
| Irritability | Walk; take slow deep breaths; do other things. |
| Trouble sleeping | Don't drink caffeine drinks in the evening; don't take naps during the day; imagine something relaxing like a favorite spot. |
| Lack of Concentration | Do something else; take a walk. |
| Tiredness | Exercise; get plenty of rest. |
| Dizziness | Sit or lie down when needed; know it will pass. |
| Headaches | Relax; take mild pain medication as needed. |

| Withdrawal Symptom | Things You Might Do |
|---|---|
| Coughing | Sip water. |
| Tightness in chest | Know it will pass. (Tightness of the chest can be a dangerous symptom under the following circumstances: |

· If it *is* severe and lasts more than three minutes,
· If the pain spreads to the jaw, neck or arms
· If you feel your heart racing
· If you experience shortness of breath, nausea or vomiting,

**Under such circumstances, you need to go to the ER for evaluation of your heart.**

| | |
|---|---|
| Constipation | Drink lots of water; eat high fiber foods like vegetables and fruits. |
| Hunger | Eat well-balanced meals; eat low-calorie snacks; drink cold water. |

For yourself and for anyone who lives with you—wife, child, parent, lover—give up cigarettes. Keep in mind that you're hurting not only yourself but also anyone else who inhales your secondhand smoke. If your spouse or partner is the smoker, show you care by urging him or her to quit—for his or her sake and yours.

Your health care provider can tell you about the products available to help you quit, such as nicotine chewing gum and patches, hypnosis and acupuncture.

Quitting is hard, so try not to get discouraged if you find it a struggle. Just keep these simple truths in mind:

- Even if you have smoked all your life, quitting will make you healthier.
- After you quit, your lungs will start healing.
- Your chance of dying of a heart attack will be 50 percent less after you quit for one year.
- Each year you don't smoke the odds get better
- After fifteen years, your chance of dying of lung cancer equals that of someone who never smoked.

Your lungs will heal. You just have to give them a chance.

You don't have to quit smoking without help. Because nicotine is recognized as highly addictive, those who have quit or are trying to quit have formed support groups similar to groups formed around other addictions, like alcohol or other drugs. Your provider or your local lung association can tell you where to find quitters support groups in your area.

For more information, contact:

The American Cancer Society
1599 Clifton Road, N. E.
Atlanta, Ga., 30329
(800) ACS-2345
Web site: http://www.cancer org.


or


American Lung Association.
1740 Broadway
NY, NY 10019
(212) 315–8700
Web site: http://www.lungusa.org


## REDUCING ALCOHOL INTAKE

Your provider may ask you to limit how much alcohol you
drink. If you belong to a social group in which people drink,
you may feel awkward at first. If you're not ready to change
your friends, hold a glass in your hand when you're with people drinking together. Here are a few examples of the many
good and healthy choices you can make about what to put in
your glass:

- Nonalcoholic beer
- Tonic water with a twist of lime
- Fruit juice

- Mineral water

If your provider thinks you can continue to drink but must cut back the amount of alcohol you drink, try having drinks that contain less alcohol, such as wine spritzers instead of a glass of wine. Instead of having two beers with your friends, have one slow beer followed by a soft drink.

If any of this is terribly hard for you, if you find it difficult or impossible to stop drinking or slow it down, get some help. *Cutting back on alcohol shouldn't be difficult for you or a big deal. If it is, you have a substance abuse problem and need help to work it out.*

## EXERCISE

Regular exercise is essential for anyone who wants to stay physically and emotionally healthy. That's as true for people with HIV as for anyone else. The kind of exercise we're talking about is different from what people do to lose weight. You shouldn't start on any weight loss program if you have HIV before speaking about it with your health care provider.

The exercise you need is simple movement! Too many African Americans aren't moving. They're "sedentary." They lie around too much, watch television too much, drive when they should have walked, and take escalators or elevators when they should have taken the stairs.

In 1997, 40 percent of adults had no leisure-time physical activity and only 15% spent at least thirty minutes in moderate physical activity, like walking. The shame is that we Black

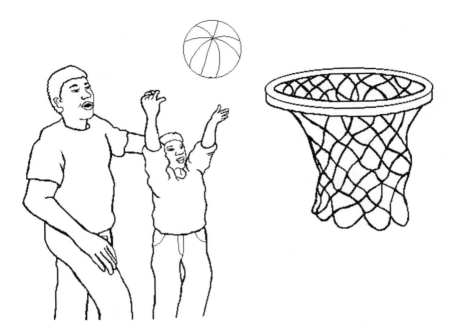

people, who have given the world so many of its greatest athletes, tend to be even less physically active than Whites. This hurts us. We're designed for walking and breathing fresh air, and when we don't get those stimulants we don't do as well.

Doctors recommend that every American engage in moderate or strenuous physical activity for at least thirty minutes at least three times a week. Some experts think we should exercise *every* day, for an hour each day. But for you, the key is to get started.

The first step is just to find the activity you do enjoy, or did enjoy, or want to be able to enjoy. It all depends on your physical condition and your taste. Some people with HIV are able to take part in strenuous sports like running, or playing basketball or tennis, or swimming. Others prefer aerobics classes, or even doing aerobics to a tape—though that keeps you indoors and alone. People who have always danced may want to continue getting their exercise by dancing. Others will enjoy walking on the street, or in a nearby park, or even, if nothing else is available or the weather's bad, a mall. Even people who are bed-ridden can sometimes do light exercise, and when they can, they feel better for it.

Exercise can be a time for socializing, if you choose a sport or an activity like team sports or dancing, or it can be something you do alone, in your own living room or outside, as a way of spending a little time by yourself. That's how it is with walking and running, too. Some people like to walk or run alone, others prefer to go out with partners or a small group.

If you can afford it (some insurance covers this), belonging to a Y or other fitness club can have advantages. People who work out are very supportive of one another. They know that what's important is the willingness to make the effort. So a club gives you a new circle of friends, who will also support you. All such clubs can be helpful in getting you started. They are trained to set up exercise programs that are just right for your needs.

*Whether you work alone or with others, the key is the same: start slowly and with your health care provider's recommendation.*

If you prefer to work out in your home, you can find workout tapes in your public library, or, if you prefer to buy one, at your corner store. Just remember to start slowly. That's where having the company of somebody else already *in* an exercise routine can be helpful.

But whether you work alone or with others, the key is the same: start slowly and with your health care provider's recommendation. If you haven't exercised in a long time, begin with a fifteen minute workout three times a week and gradually build up to thirty minutes by the end of the first month. Go at an easy pace—you shouldn't be panting and sweating profusely. If you are, you are working too hard. Make this an enjoyable experience, one that you can look forward to.

Walking is ideal exercise. It costs little, and everyone can find someplace to walk, even if it's only the couple of blocks to the grocery store and back. If you take up walking as your exercise, all you need is a pair of good walking shoes and clothing that suits the weather. In really bad weather or if you want to get away from the neighborhood, you can walk around a mall. A lot of people get their exercise that way, especially in the winter.

Like everything else, an exercise routine is something you can get into gradually. Maybe for the first week, just go to the corner and back. Do that three times. On the second week, you'll want to try once around the block. Or maybe on the third. You set the pace. If you keep at it, at a modest level, after a while you'll feel better and stronger and ready for more.

Regular exercise makes its benefits obvious after only a few weeks. People who exercise sleep better, have more energy, and enjoy meals more. Don't take my word for it. Try it. It works!

Once you have gotten into a regular exercise routine, you'll start looking for other ways to stretch your legs. You'll prefer to walk those extra two blocks to work, or to park at the far end of the parking lot and take the stairs instead of the elevator. You'll enjoy walking to do your errands. That way you can turn an obligation into a pleasure, listen to the birds sing, exchange some words with a friend on the street, breathe the air, feel the muscles in your legs, swing your arms—know you're alive.

In the old days people had no choice but to exercise. Work was exercise, transportation was exercise, getting food was exercise—maybe too much of a good thing. But today, for many of us, sedentary lifestyles make it difficult to stay in shape. Even our jobs, often, don't require much physical work, and so much of modern technology—cars, computers, and televisions—seem designed to make us less active.

You just have to be conscious of those pressures, and know that moving less isn't in your best interest. Get your exercise, at whatever level feels comfortable for you and is OK with your provider.

## EATING WELL

Eating is one of the joys of life. And eating well brings joy and strength to our bodies. Your body needs plenty of vitamins and minerals to keep fighting HIV. The HIV is going after your CD4 cells and killing them. Your body is countering this by making extra CD4 cells. Your body makes cells and body tissues from the protein, vitamins and minerals you eat. So to fight the good fight against HIV, you have to eat well.

### To Increase your Appetite

At some point during your HIV or, more likely, during your treatment, you may lose your appetite. If this happens, tell your health care provider so you can make sure it is not a sign of an infection or of the HIV getting worse.

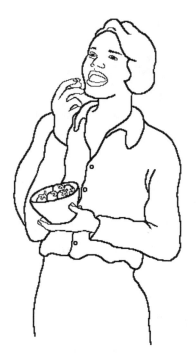

If you have a bad taste in your mouth, brush your teeth more often or gargle with lightly salted water. Some people recommend sucking on a lemon wedge before eating to get rid of a metallic taste sometimes caused by the medications.

It's important that you eat regular healthy meals, so eat foods that you like and that are good for you.

To make food more enticing, spice it up:

- Add more garlic and strong spices
- Marinate meats or tofu in natural teriyaki sauce or Italian dressing
- Cook meats or tofu with fruits or sauces (as, for example, pineapple or orange chicken)

## A Wholesome Diet

A wholesome diet contains the following elements:

- Hearty breads and cereals
- Low-fat proteins like broiled fish and chicken
- Fresh fruits and fresh green vegetables
- Whole grains, like oats, or brown rice, bulgur or kasha
- Low-salt foods
- Low-sugar foods

Breads and whole grain cereals give us fiber, which may help to lower blood sugar and blood fat levels, and which can help keep us regular. Foods high in fiber include bran cereals, cooked beans and peas, whole-grain bread, fruits and vegetables.

Remember that high fats lead to heart disease and clogged arteries. This is especially important to the HIV patient, because a long-term side effect of certain drugs is to elevate cholesterol and triglycerides (fats) in the blood. If you are taking protease inhibitors, you will need to work out with your provider a diet that will keep cholesterol and triglycerides from building up in your arteries.

Consuming less salt is important because of the epidemic rates of high blood pressure among Black people. For some people, at least, there is a clear relationship between salt and the danger of stroke and kidney disease. The last thing you need is another disease! Cutting back on salt may cut your risk of high blood pressure.

Many vitamins and minerals are found in fresh vegetables and fruits. Those with the brightest colors tend to have more nutrients: dark green lettuce, collards and greens, broccoli, carrots, oranges and bananas, for example. If you are not already eating fresh foods, start slowly and work up to a diet that includes salads, fresh fruits and steamed or lightly fried vegetables.

Candy, cookies, soda, cakes and desserts usually have a lot of calories, fat, sugar and salt, but are low in vitamins and minerals. That's why sweets are called "empty calories." These foods should be eaten only occasionally, not as part of a regular diet.

Too often, people fill up on a bag of cookies, which supplies calories but provides none of the vitamins and minerals our bodies crave and need. We were designed to eat fresh fruit, fruit juice and real foods, not candy and soda. Over time, a diet that relies on cookies and sweets every day deprives a person of necessary vitamins and minerals and can lead to deficiencies.

*Over time, a diet that relies on cookies and sweets every day deprives a person of necessary vitamins and minerals and can lead to deficiencies.*

Soda pop needs special mention because it's especially bad for us. It is packed with sugar and calories and phosphorus. The phosphorus interferes with our ability to absorb calcium, the mineral that makes our teeth and bones. That loss is particularly hard on women, who generally do not get enough calcium. Drink soda and you will be filled up—but not with the kind of food your body needs. (All sweets are very hard on teeth, too, especially children's teeth.)

If you want to cut back on eating sweets, start by getting them out of the house. Avoid any sweet that takes control over you, that gives you cravings so you are not satisfied and eat more than a reasonable portion. With other sweets, try cutting back gradually. For a few weeks, cut out the cookies you eat every afternoon but let yourself have the piece of pie after dinner. Then, have the piece of pie three nights a week instead of every night. After a couple weeks, limit the pie to one special night a week. You will enjoy it more, too. Substitute fruit, fruit juice, low-sodium vegetable juice, dried fruits and whole-grain crackers for sweets.

You'll be surprised at how easy it is to cut back on sweets if you are exercising regularly. Exercising has a way of "tuning up" the body. Your tastes may change as you exercise, so that you begin to seek out the foods your body needs, like fruits and whole grains, and fresh vegetables.

Many experts recommend that people with HIV eat yogurt with live acidophilus cultures. The acidophilus is similar to the healthy bacteria found in our intestines. When there is plenty of it, we tend to have fewer GI upsets and bouts with yeast overgrowth. When you choose yogurt, check the sell-by date to make sure it is fresh, and choose brands that have live acidophilus cultures.

While you may want to add new foods to your diet, check with your health care provider before doing so. Certain foods, such as grapefruit, may interact with drugs you are taking to fight your HIV or its related diseases. What you need to know is if there are special dietary restrictions on the drugs in your particular cocktail. For example, Didanosine or Indinavir should be taken on an empty stomach, while others, like Efavirinz,® should not be taken after high-fat meals, because fat affects its absorption. Still others, like Nelfinavir,® will favorably increase its absorption with a fatty meal. You must take all protease inhibitors, too, with food.

## SWITCHING TO A HEALTHY DIET

If you're like many Americans today, your diet depends a lot on fast food, snacks and preprepared food that you just have to stick in the oven or microwave. We eat this stuff because it fits into our busy lives. But these foods tend to be loaded with extra, unnecessary calories, have high amounts of bad fat, sugar and salt. These aren't the kinds of substances that fuel our body in its fight against HIV. Our body craves good carbohydrates, like oatmeal and whole grain breads, lean meats and fish and fresh fruits and vegetables.

Even the food we associate with being Black in this country can be a problem when we're fighting to keep the body strong. Foods such as salty collard greens, smoked pork, ribs, fried chicken and macaroni and cheese, made like Mama made them, can be high in fat and calories, as well as salt.

These foods are part of our tradition, and few of us want to give them up. The good news is, you don't have to. Just learn to like them when they're *not* fried and when they're cooked with less salt, or none. Your nutritionist can suggest some tasty salt substitutes. The nutritionist may also recommend that you make your macaroni and cheese with low-fat cheese, and cook your greens with no lard (use vegetable oil instead), and a lot less salt.

You have other help in addition to your nutritionists. Some local AIDS advocacy organizations serve free or low-cost healthy lunches and dinners for people with HIV. If you cook

# FAT, CHOLESTEROL, CALORIES AND SODIUM CONTENT IN JUNK FOODS

| Snack (1 ounce | Saturated Fat (grams) | Cholesterol (mgs) | Total Fat (grams) | Calories from Fat (%) | Total Calories | Sodium (mgs) |
|---|---|---|---|---|---|---|
| Pretzels, salted (1 oz. is about 5 twists, 3 1/4 x 2 1/4 x 1/4 in.) | 0.2 | 0 | 1.0 | 8 | 108 | 486 |
| Popcorn, air popped without salt (1 oz. is about 3 1/2 cups) | 0.2 | 0 | 1.2 | 10 | 108 | 1 |
| Tortilla chips, lower fat (light) nacho flavor | 0.8 | 1 | 4.3 | 31 | 126 | 284 |
| Corn Chips | 1.3 | 0 | 9.5 | 56 | 153 | 179 |
| Popcorn, popped with oil and salt (1 oz. is about 2 1/2 cups) | 1.4 | 0 | 8.0 | 51 | 142 | 251 |
| Tortilla chips, nacho flavor | 1.4 | 1 | 7.3 | 47 | 141 | 201 |
| Trail mix (1 oz. is about 1/5 cups | 1.6 | 0 | 8.3 | 57 | 131 | 65 |
| Potato chips | 3.1 | 0 | 9.8 | 58 | 152 | 168 |

Reprinted from NIHLBI, "Step by Step: Eating to Lower Your Blood Cholesterol" (February 1999), p. 10.

at home, you'll find excellent low-fat soul food recipes in *The Heart of the Matter: The African American's Guide to Heart Disease, Heart Treatment, and Heart Wellness*, by Hilton M. Hudson , M.D. and Herbert Stern, Ph.D. (Roscoe, IL: Hilton Publishing Company, 2000)

Your new diet will mean three meals a day. Each meal will include:

- One protein food, such as dairy, meat, fish or eggs
- One grain, such as bread or oatmeal or cornmeal
- One or two servings of vegetables and fruits.

Healthy snacks, especially of fresh fruit, yogurt, whole grain crackers and nuts are just fine. But try not to eat potato chips, corn chips or other junk foods. They give you a lot of salt, a lot of fat, and not enough vitamins and minerals. They take away your appetite for the good foods you need.

Here are examples of what meals might look like under your new, healthier diet:

- Breakfast: oatmeal with milk; a glass of orange, apple or prune juice; and a banana.
- Lunch: a salad and a sandwich of whole wheat bread with ham, tuna fish, chicken breast or peanut butter, followed by a piece of fruit and a cup of yogurt
- Dinner: a salad, steamed broccoli or spinach, and macaroni and low-fat cheese, or broiled, skinless chicken breast, followed by fresh fruit, or canned fruit with no sugar added

# CHOOSE A HEALTHIER SNACK

Snack on...

Air-popped popcorn with no butter, unsalted pretzels
Hard candy, jelly beans
Bagels, raisin toast or English muffins with margarine or jelly
Low-fat cookies (such as fig bars, vanilla wafers, gingersnaps)
Fruits, vegetables
Fruit juices and drinks
Frozen yogurt, sherbet, ice pops

Instead of...

Popcorn with butter
Chocolate bars
Doughnuts, Danish pastry
Cake, cookies, brownies
Milk shakes, eggnogs, floats
Ice cream

Reprinted from National Institute of Health: E*at Right to Lower Your High Blood Cholesterol*, March 1992.

Make changes to your diet slowly. For example, start by substituting whole wheat bread for white bread and wait a week before making another food change. Or add yogurt to your diet by having a bowl once a day as a snack. Don't introduce any other foods until the next week.

Go slowly, because changing your diet too quickly can

upset your digestive system. Besides, the changes you stay with are usually the slow, steady ones. Start off in the right frame of mind. You don't have to stop eating your favorite foods. That would be to give up a great source of comfort. Just make your changes slowly and steadily, giving yourself a chance to take in new foods and flavors that are also healthier for you.

## A WORD ABOUT SALT

Salty foods can be deadly. For some people, they contribute to hypertension and even stroke. Cutting back on the amount of salt you eat is a way of doing yourself a big favor.

The official recommendation is that adults eat no more than 2,400 milligrams (mgs.) of salt per day. But American food manufacturers love salt—it is in everything, even cookies—so most Americans consume much more than 2,400 mgs. per day. If you want to reduce the amount of salt you eat each day, you have to be very, very careful about what you eat.

High salt content is found in some unexpected products, like grocery store cakes and cookies. Read the labels. Avoid junk food, fast food, and prepared food as much as you can. Again, the rule holds: take it slow, but take it!

Here's an example of what we're talking about. A Burger King Double Whopper™ with cheese provides 1,460 mgs. of salt. If you add fries, you are over 2,400 mgs. If you eat a dessert, you will be way above 2,400! And fast food fried chicken is no different. It's so tasty. But part of what makes it so is the extraordinary amount of salt in the "secret recipe" bread coating. Not to mention the gobs of saturated fat and high amount of calories.

At first it may be hard to give up junk foods. Avoid these and other salty foods for two months, then treat yourself to a big fried chicken meal, and you may be disgusted. It will taste too salty! If you avoid salt, your taste buds will change. They will become more sensitive to salt, the way they were when you were a child. Ask anyone on a low-salt diet and that person will tell you the same thing: as he or she cut down on salt, the taste buds woke up to the rich but subtler tastes of the food itself.

Fast foods can be tempting because they seem to be a good bargain. The advertising, aimed especially at Black Americans, wants to make you think that these fast foods go along with "family values." Don't you believe it! These foods were designed to make profit, not to nourish and strengthen your body. These foods rob us of our health. They're not even cheap When you realize that your bad health may be part of the cost.

## NO FRYING

Heavily fried foods taste delicious but they are very unhealthy. They add a huge amount of unnecessary calories, salt and fat, and sometimes toxins as well. Oils for deep-frying change in chemical composition when they are used more than once, as is often the case at fast food restaurants. The oil changes so much that our bodies treat it as a toxic substance.

For these and other reasons, it is a good idea to cut back on deep-fried foods, like fast-food chicken and burgers. Such foods should be eaten as a very special treat (if you still have any desire for them).

The best way, the most economical way, and the safest way to know what you're eating is to cook your meals at home.

Instead of frying, learn to steam, bake, and microwave, adding a small amount of safflower, canola or olive oil when needed.

Butter and lard should be used sparingly. Animal fats tend to speed clogging of the arteries. We want to go in the other direction, to eat and live in ways that will give our hearts and blood vessels the chance to function properly.

## VITAMINS AND ALTERNATIVE TREATMENTS

Your provider may recommend vitamin supplements. Or you might have heard from friends or an advocacy group about a good mix of vitamins to try. This is fine, but run it by your health care provider first, especially with herbal and other supplements. Some of these mixtures are powerful. Your provider needs to know what you are taking in case any of the items interact with drugs he or she has prescribed. Over-the-counter herbs, like Saint-John's-wort (for mood elevation) interacts with ARVs, often requiring a dosage adjustment.

# CHAPTER 13

# HIV, STRESS AND STRESS RELIEF

To have HIV or love someone who has it is to be under great stress. Nobody knows that better than you. Maybe you're the sort of person who believes a man or woman must handle stress without any outside help, lest you show weakness. It doesn't have to be like that. If you have HIV you may well have more than you can handle, yet, in order to stay well, you *must* handle it. That's why you need to organize yourself and others into a work team. You need medical assistance, certainly, but you also should have support for *all* your needs, social and emotional.

The main goal of this chapter is to encourage you to do just that: see a counselor, your health care provider or social worker or join a support group to talk out the stress that you are feeling. Talking it out with someone who can listen deeply will give you relief and show you ways to reduce not only the stress that comes from having HIV but also the stress that comes from normal living.

*Integrating the new realities that being HIV-positive presents is a process of reprioritizing one's life. In my experience, everyone needs help in defining this new self-perception.*

It doesn't work to hold stress inside. Fears and anger come out when you least want them to, sometimes in ways that can leave you out of control. That is why your provider has probably encouraged you to see a counselor, speak with a social worker, or join a support group. This is nothing to be ashamed of or embarrassed about. HIV is a serious disease that carries with it heaps of social and personal baggage. Fear, anger, the sense of being overwhelmed by new responsibilities—no human being can be expected to carry this load alone. Integrating the new realities that being HIV-positive presents is a process of reprioritizing one's life. In my experience, everyone needs help in defining this new self-perception.

You don't have to be driven over the edge of despair by HIV and its stress. Resources are available to help you continue *living* with HIV. But first you need to know a few things about stress.

## WHAT HAPPENS IN OUR BODIES DURING STRESS

Stress is one of the body's emergency systems. During stress, blood is sent away from the stomach and out to the arms, legs and brain. It drives us to run, fight or think about how to save ourselves. Stress is an alarm to the body to use all its resources for self-preservation. When stress becomes a full-time process, it does damage. It's like driving all the time with the pedal on the metal.

Stress can harm your body by:

- Decreasing blood flow to the stomach, which can lead to ulcers
- Over-stimulating the adrenal gland's secretion of cortisol, a chemical that can be toxic to the gland in the heavy doses caused by stress
- Making the body less able to absorb glucose, the simple sugar the body normally uses as fuel, leading to diabetes

Stress also has strong influence on how high your CD4 counts are, how fast they go down, and how you feel in general. Constant stress will wear you down faster. It can bring on AIDS quicker.

Your immune system is stronger and your CD4 cells work better when you are relaxed. When people are stressed, whether they have HIV or not, their CD4 counts drop for a period and they are more vulnerable to illness and infec-

*Constant stress will wear you down faster. It can bring on AIDS quicker.*

tion. According to a study made at Carnegie Mellon University, people experiencing high stress were twice as likely to get colds. That suggests their immune systems were weakened. Today, researchers are exploring the details of how this works.

But you don't need to be a researcher to know that stress works against you. Stress can push you to smoke and drink more, to fall back into doing drugs, to miss sleep and exercise—in short, to do all the things that will weaken the immune system even further. Don't let that happen to you.

You can learn new, healthier and more satisfying ways to handle stress. Your job is to be open to them.

## STRESS AND DEPRESSION

Chronic stress (stress that we have all the time) hurts us emotionally even as it hurts us physically. Signs of chronic stress include:

- Not sleeping well
- Using drugs or drinking heavily
- Frequent, sudden, angry outbursts
- Withdrawing from those around you
- Depression
- Unexplained fatigue
- Compulsive sex
- Feeling worthless
- Feeling alone all the time, even with friends and family
- Dark thoughts, including suicide

Depression is common among people with HIV, particularly those who are newly diagnosed. Depression can also build up when we are faced over and over again with stress and the feeling of isolation that goes with it, to the point that we just can't cope anymore and feel helplessly trapped. The inability to cope causes feelings of worthlessness, and these feelings make the whole thing worse. Often, it's under the pressures of stress and depression that a person turns to drugs, alcohol, stimulants or even food addiction. Even violence or acts that hurt oneself can result from stress.

In the African American community, depression tends to be overlooked and under-reported—in part because it's often seen as a sign of weakness or a sign that the victim has lost faith in life itself, and in part because of the terrible impact of poverty and lack of knowledge that can accompany it in the Black community.

That's especially unfortunate because today there are a number of ways, ranging from counseling to medication, to treat depression effectively. There is no reason that we in the community should not make use of emotional health resources that the White community takes for granted. If you or someone you know shows symptoms of depression, call the nurse for help. Available treatments, including counseling and medication, can help you feel better. Don't let your stress and depression go unattended. Your health care provider, counselor, social worker or support group can guide you to the help you need.

Human beings are not built to go through life in a state of perpetual anxiety, anger or fear. We were made to be happy, relaxed and thoughtful, with only occasional bouts of worry and anger. That's the zone where we feel loving, where we value ourselves and where we can best live productive lives.

People diagnosed with HIV can live a reasonably stress-free life if they pay attention to the signs and know how to deal with them. Take a step in the right direction by checking yourself against the signs of chronic stress above. Do any of these ring true with you? If so, those bad feelings may contribute to more rapid progression of your HIV.

You will have a better chance of keeping your CD4 count

up and maintaining a healthy immune response if you take a little time to identify and eliminate the stress in your life. Not to do so is to put your mental as well as your physical health at risk. Severe stress can turn into chronic depression, a state in which a person is very sad and unmotivated and may have feelings of suicide. You don't want to go there.

## STRESS AND GRIEF

Grief is a form of stress that needs special attention. You may experience grief upon learning you are HIV-positive because of the fear that you won't live as long as you should. Yes, we can grieve for ourselves, and the lost life in us. Grief may also come from the deaths of those around you who succumbed to AIDS, drugs, violence or old age. Sometimes, just to look around is more than we can bear.

It's not just in fairy tales that people die of broken hearts. In real life, too, grief and loss and isolation can harm you deeply. The remedy is to share your grief. Share it with friends, counselors or your support group. Find safe places where you can say how you feel, and it will fall on kind and sympathetic ears. At the same time, take the time you need with your grief. Honest grieving isn't the same as depression. It's a way of feeling pain we must feel before we can heal and go on.

So don't expect grief to go away overnight. It's a common but unrealistic belief that grief should go away after a week or two. Healing comes in its own time. It can take months, or years, and, grief, by its nature, has periods of great intensity. But healing comes faster to those who actively acknowledge grief and depression in their lives.

Even while you are grieving, you can look for opportunities to heal and renew your engagement in life and people. Giving to others, even in small ways, helps you work through your grief. Such human contact shows you that life is good and continuous. Such contact can be as simple as hearing a child laugh, or watching a dog at play. Let others touch your loss and help you heal. We aren't meant to be in this world alone.

If you are a recovering addict, you've already begun to learn ways to come out of your isolation. Being very self-absorbed, you became isolated. What was uppermost in your mind was getting drugs or alcohol for yourself. You neglected the people you love and who love you.

Being free of addiction means looking outside of yourself and sometimes tending to the needs of others. Opening yourself up to others is good for your health! The good, the generous and the happy live longer than the hostile and self-absorbed. They also have a better time.

## AFRICAN AMERICANS AND STRESS

Because African Americans are terribly familiar with the feeling of social isolation, we experience more than our share of stress. As a legacy of the sustained impact of slavery, racism and discrimination are still embedded in the very fabric of our workplaces, schools and the places in which we do business. Racism informs and molds our self-images, for better and for worse. It often makes us try harder. But, at the same time, under the conditions of racism, it's difficult to know if your boss is giving you a hard time because of your performance or because of your skin color.

As African Americans, we are constantly obliged to filter other people's messages that challenge our credibility, competency and intelligence. That's why we all need to learn at very early ages not to allow a message of inferiority to become part of our self-perception.

In everyday life, many of us feel challenged every time we leave the house. When you walk into a well-lit department store at noon to purchase socks for your children, and the woman standing in front of you clutches her purse close to her, is it because she's nervous and would do this when anyone came up behind her, or because you are Black? In these cases what makes for chronic stress isn't the certainty that you are being met with bigotry. It's the uncertainty.

Counseling can do a lot to relieve stress, and to teach you how to manage what you can't relieve. (That's just one more reason why it's so important for you to keep up counseling or a support group at least once a week.) But counseling works only when you work. A most effective way to make yourself work is to give yourself goals.

If you have been an addict and are not using now, your life is on the mend. But you may not have had goals or dreams for quite some time. You left them behind when you gave up your life for drugs or alcohol.

You can have goals again if you know how to make use of the support available. Sure, having goals means wanting something, and wanting carries risk with it. But counselors and support groups can help you through the fear that may come up when you see that your life can be in your own hands again. With the right kind of help and support, you can achieve your goals. Start small, one day at a time. The more small goals you accomplish, the more courage you will have for the big goals.

It's in your power to be engaged in life, make positive decisions that benefit you and your loved ones, and maintain confidence in the future.

## STAYING CONNECTED

An underlying theme of this chapter is that you need to stay connected with other human beings in your world. That may take positive effort. Often, just after being diagnosed, people feel terribly isolated by their own fear that they will have to face their hard struggle alone.

Once again, this can be worse for African Americans. We often face feelings of social isolation when we are outside our home communities, however we define them—our neighborhoods, churches, families and best friends. That already familiar feeling of social isolation may be heightened with a diagnosis of HIV and all of the societal trappings that the diagnosis brings.

The danger here is that this feeling of desperate isolation can keep you from seeking the help you need. Black people

*You need to stay connected with other human beings in your world. That may take positive effort. Often, just after being diagnosed, people feel terribly isolated by their own fear that they will have to face their hard struggle alone.*

who have felt the sting of racism when they moved outside home communities may be hesitant to look for help, fearing they must face again the same kind of situation that's so often made them feel bad before.

You don't have to feel isolated—not even by racism. On a personal level, if not on a political one, the reality is less important than how you feel about it. Yes, you are a Black American who has HIV. But you are also a human being, entitled to the best help that can be provided to those in desperate need. Often, with just a phone call, you'll find people out there who are trained and eager to help.

Just remember that it's your job to set the ball rolling, by reaching out to your church, your good friends and family, your counselor, your support group. Other people will help you laugh and cry your way through your diagnosis, your treatments, and the challenges ahead. They'll let you blow off steam safely, and they'll provide companionship, and maybe advice if you ask for it. They'll lend a hand. Don't try to make it without support. You're just rigging the odds against yourself.

The beautiful thing is that while you are serving your own needs by attending a group meeting, you'll also be helping others. At first, you'll feel needy, hungry for support. But after you've been engaged with the group a while, you will find opportunities to give back to someone more needy than you. This give and take is what makes human beings realize that they are not alone and that we all are in need.

Sometimes, curing our isolation means renewing contact with family and friends. For the person who has felt isolated, and who may in fact cut himself or herself off, renewing contact may be difficult. Begin by just listening to your own common sense. We weren't made to be alone. Whatever it takes, we must do what we can to connect with people. Even pets can help, in the way they respond to us and in the way we care for them.

You may already have what you need around you. But if you don't, don't just wait to see if it will appear. Reach out to people. Create the human solidarity we all need to hold us up in the hard times.

## TWELVE STEPS

We highly recommend twelve-step programs such as that run by Alcoholics Anonymous, which is designed to help us kick bad habits and heal us of the shame that plunged us into dependency in the first place. The theory behind twelve steps is that by admitting where we have been with our addictions, and the damage we have inflicted on those closest to us, we begin to move toward acceptance of the good and the bad in ourselves. Only when we've learned to face ourselves can true healing begin. Twelve-step programs help us learn by creating a close, supportive atmosphere, a kind of nest where healing can take place. Many people have dropped their addictions and stayed free of them through twelve-step programs.

## SUPPORT GROUPS

In a support group you can share your most painful feelings of shame, guilt and stress without losing face. And listening to the moving and sometimes heroic stories of others can help you put your own situation in perspective.

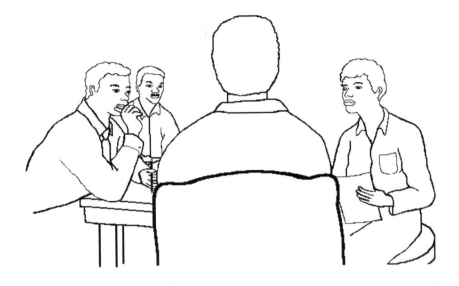

These days, support groups are available to almost everyone. Many find that being in a protected space where you can
laugh and cry freely about having HIV is good medicine. For
people who have let shame and powerlessness isolate them,
joining a support group can begin a return to the social world.
(See the Resource section for how to find support groups.)

## LEARNING TO HAVE MORE OF THE GOOD DAYS

The uncertainties that come from living with HIV on a day-
to-day basis can cause stress. If your CD4 count is high right
now, you know that at some point it may drop and you will
begin taking antiretrovirals. If your CD4 count is low already,
you may be worried that you won't remain well. In either case,
you will have good days, but you will also have bad days when
it's hard for you to keep your courage up.

So look ahead. Don't wait until that day when you learn that your CD4 count has dropped to 200 to turn to other human beings. Don't wait until you're desperate. For some people, a trusted friend can help. For other people, it's an HIV or support group. Still others find what they need in prayer or Bible groups that pray or read the Bible, or in meditation groups that meditate together. The important thing is that you have regular, reliable contact with a person or a group that gives you the blessings of a nonjudgmental listener and steady encouragement to draw upon. In the strength of others, you'll find strength to go on.

Prayer groups and Bible reading, and meditation practice can help bring you in touch with what twelve-step programs simply call "a higher power." Many people have drawn great strength by putting their lives in touch with a larger destiny, and doing so with the companionship of others.

Any method that works for you opens a channel of hope. And there's also a medical ground for hope. Today, treatments are available to you that ten years ago would have seemed miraculous. Who knows what tomorrow will bring?

To sum up, being diagnosed with HIV, sticking to the treatment, going through the ups and downs, can be very stressful. So is the guilt of possibly having passed on the virus to others. But life with HIV is not one long downer. There will be good days when HIV is not at the center of your life. You'll have more of those good days once you understand that you've done things that resulted in your becoming HIV-positive. Now, as a result, you must remain in medical care for the rest of your life. That's the stark fact and you can't change it. Once you've accepted it, make the best of it, by drawing on the new resources you'll discover in yourself, and on the help of family and friends and community workers who are dedicated to helping you get along as well as you can. In this way, you will learn to re-engage in life.

Virtually all my patients get to the point where the good days by far outnumber the bad. It is a process to get there, but the goal is achievable.

## STRESS RELIEF

You know the powerful saying: "The day we did things right was the day we stood up to fight. Keep your eyes on the prize and hold on." In talking about stress relief, the prize isn't to eliminate the causes of stress. They're part of life, and certainly part of the life of someone with HIV. To some extent they're beyond our control. Stuff happens, to paraphrase the bumper sticker. Big bills come in, somebody loses a job, your CD4 count drops although you've been doing everything right.

The prize is learning how to cope—that is learning to reject negative ways of coping with stress and developing positive ones. You've probably got a friend or neighbor like our friend Ned. Often, his troubles seem worse than ours are, but he always seems to handle them. You don't see him worrying all the time, as some of us do, or snapping at the people he loves. He isn't over-eager for his afternoon beer. He seems to start each day not with dread but with enthusiasm. Ned has learned how to cope.

Ned has learned, and you can also learn, to have a certain frame of mind, a healthy realistic view of life. Such a view realizes that life is like a roller coaster. There are ups and downs, sharp, unexpected turns, dips and rises. People like Ned have learned to enjoy the ride. What works for him is maintaining so strong an appreciation of the good things in his life that, when something bad happens, he can look at it through the lens of what's good. He doesn't see the glass as half empty, but as half full.

There's a lot to be said for the state of mind that Ned has achieved, not the least of which is that he's doing the right thing for his immune system. You may feel that Ned is one of the lucky ones, born knowing how to manage their stress, so that it rolls off them like soft rain. But lots of people—and you can be one—have *learned* what they need to know. The trick is easier to describe than it is to perform: just learn how to transform stress, and even fear, into exceptional performance. People like Ned have learned to take the so-called "negative" feelings of fear, anxiety or anger as fuel to make necessary changes in their lives or relationships. They've learned to take lessons from bad situations, and in that way to change them.

Let's take anger as an example. For some of us, constant anger makes a lot of trouble. It drives away loved ones; it may hurt us on the job. It makes us do crazy, self-destructive things and to feel, at the time we're doing them, that we just don't give a damn.

Anger can have a thousand sources. It may go back to old wounds—something that happened, or didn't happen, when you were a kid. It may be the result of racism, the real racism that you experience day to day. Or it may be a sign that you are trapped in an unfair situation—perhaps a dead-end job or a relationship in which the other person takes more than they give. Or it may be that you're not willing to accept the facts of your situation, like the fact that you have HIV.

The first step in coping with anger is to think about why you are feeling it. By sharing your thoughts with a counselor or trusted friend, you can change anger into a plan: make a change in the situation or turn to a healthy way to relieve the stress. The first time you work out a plan with your provider for your treatment, you've taken a major step in relieving your stress. Sure, problems can seem so big that any solution or relief seems impossible. But no matter what your situation is, there are better and worse ways of handling it. With the help of other people, you can choose the better way.

## Identify the Stress

*Your counselor, your friends and your support groups can be of great help, but coping with stress also means acting to help yourself.* Coping with any problem starts with identifying it. But that's not always as easy as it sounds. If you've been living in stress for a long time, it's like the air you breathe. You're used to it. It's like anger itself. It just happens, as if without your say-so.

Your first job is to open up a little space between you and the stress. You begin doing that by identifying when and why you are stressed.

A diagnosis of being HIV-positive brings new stresses on top of the old ones:

- Maybe you fear telling people about your HIV, or about being gay, bisexual, transgender or a drug user.

- Maybe what scares you is juggling the paperwork associated with your medical bills, or having to take time
off from your job in order to see the provider.
- Maybe you are living with a friend or spouse who,
unlike you, is not HIV-positive, and your loved one is
terribly worried, too, about you and maybe about his or
her own health. (In such a case, you may want to see a
counselor together.)

Breaking the news to loved ones can be a big source of
worry. But if you work at it, you can turn that worry into a
course of action. Let's say you're afraid your mother will react
badly to the news. Talk it over with a member of the family,
somebody who cares about your mother and cares about you.
Often, in such conversations, a key to the situation becomes
clear. In this case, that key is how to tell your mother calmly
and honestly who you are, in a way that does not cause a rift
between you. Usually in matters like these, if there's a will,
there's a way.

When you are living with your stress, you'll find that some
days are worse than others. Say, you've just learned that your
CD4 count has dropped or that you have an infection. News
like that and its aftermath could put people you into an emotional state of permanent crisis. A state like that is exactly
what you don't need.

When you're hit with bad news, take a deep breath. Think
about all the efforts you've made already, and all the progress.
Remind yourself that, with proper treatment, you can get
through this crisis. And, of course, talking this out with a
counselor or a friend can bring you relief. The key to stress

management, if you're HIV-positive, is to anticipate the need and know how to find the help.

Another thing you should know about stress is that you need to cut yourself a little slack. There will be days when you can't point to any one thing that happened; you just came home at the end of the day "stressed out," and now you're acting like a little kid, unreasonable. You hate having HIV and you just don't want to deal with it.

You're entitled to these feelings. By letting yourself experience them, you put yourself in touch with the deeper layers of your feeling. Take such feelings to your counselor. He or she can help you find healing in that place deep inside you.

*The key to stress management, if you're HIV-positive, is to anticipate the need and know how to find the help*

On your own and with the help of a counselor or a support group, your job is to identify the deep sources of your stress, sources over which you can have some control. Usually, "control" means learning to look at a problem from a new angle that lets you see a solution. The solution is always simple: facing an unpleasant fact and finding positive ways to work with it. Such work requires patience and determination. But if you keep at it, before long you'll experience the satisfaction that comes to those who keep the faith in their ability to live positive lives.

### Sleep

Coping with stress, like coping with ordinary life, means getting enough sleep. If we go without adequate sleep for very long, most of us get cranky and less able to concentrate. If you have HIV, the anger and moodiness that comes from sleeplessness can make you more vulnerable to your HIV and to other infections.

Regulating sleep means avoiding stimulants like alcohol, caffeine and nicotine, especially the closer you get to your bedtime. All of them can disrupt sleep. Some people don't drink coffee or soda after 3 P.M. or earlier. This is what works for them. Find out what works for you.

There are also positive things you can do. Develop good habits for getting ready to sleep. That means not getting overstimulated, and taking deliberate steps to soothe yourself.

If you watch a violent movie before going to bed, you're not likely to slip easily into sleep. It's much better to read something that soothes or even bores you, or to listen to mellow music.

Once in bed, remove the obvious obstacles to sleep. Use earplugs to eliminate annoying noise. Relax your body methodically, tensing and then relaxing muscles—start with your feet, then gradually move up your legs, to the trunk of your body, your chest, neck, jaw, cheeks and brow. Do it a few times if necessary. It works.

Paying attention to your breathing can also help. Try to steady and slow it. Give attention to your breath. When your mind wanders, bring it back, gently, to the breath.

If none of this helps, bring your problem to your counselor or support group and tell your health care provider. Maybe a medication you are taking is interfering with your sleep. You may be depressed. Or maybe there is some issue that you aren't

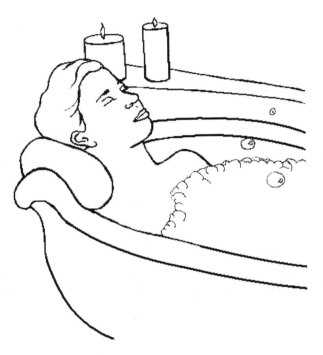

consciously aware of that is troubling you that you can bring to the surface and work out with the help of your counselor.

Sleeplessness is like many problems: there are better and worse ways of dealing with it. By choosing the better ones, you may soon find that the problem is under control. You need your sleep. Your body needs it to mend. Your spirit needs it for the same reasons.

## Exercise

Being ill isn't necessarily a reason not to exercise. You're going to have good days, and even on the bad ones, light exercise can be a way of pushing back. Exercise takes energy, yes, but it gives more than it takes. So if you can, get out of the house, walk around. Walking not only gives you exercise, it gets you out and about and keeps you from brooding.

If you can't get out, ask your health care provider to prescribe light exercise you can do at home. Don't let yourself get sedentary if you can help it. Regular exercise will make you feel better. It will also help you feel that you are taking control of your life.

## CONCLUSION

In this book I've looked at a wide range of issues and concerns that face African American individuals and communities who wish to work actively against HIV. The ground floor of the discussion is understanding the natural history of HIV, its movement through our community and its destructive impact on your immune function. From this foundation, I have tried to develop a rational, nonjudgmental strategy that would apply to a range of human experience, knowing that not everything will be useful to all readers, but trying to be comprehensive in the solutions offered.

Our understanding of HIV is growing fast, and it requires constant vigilance on everyone's part to keep up with the new information. Your health care provider is responsible for keeping abreast of this information and making it part of your treatment plan. Your provider can best do this through open dialogue with you. That dialogue will have its starts and stops, and, sometimes, even changes in direction. The key here is that the dialogue should be informed and honest, and continually assess whether the treatment is meeting *your* needs.

HIV has been in our community for a long time. We can start changing this situation, today, by combining our efforts to stop the spread of this epidemic and by removing the barriers that keep our brothers and sisters from finding and getting the care we deserve.

# RESOURCES

## 1. WHERE TO GET TESTED FOR AIDS:

If you or a friend wants to get a free, confidential test for HIV and you don't know where to go, call the National AIDS Hotline: 1-800-342-2437.

## 2. FOR INFORMATION ABOUT AFRICAN AMERICANS AND AIDS

Log onto the site of the U.S. Office of Minority Health Research, www.omhr.gov/omh/AIDS.

Another site to look at is the National Minority AIDS Coalition, which strives to develop leadership among communities of color about HIV. Log onto the website www.nmac.org.

The National AIDS Treatment Advocacy Project posts summaries of talks by AIDS experts concerning HIV and African Americans. Log on at: www.natp.org.

The U.S. Centers for Disease Control gathers statistics about the spread of HIV in different populations. You can call them for written information: 1-800-342-AIDS or log on to its website: www.cdc.gov/hiv.

The website, www.blackhealthnetwork.com, also has information about African Americans and HIV.

For information on being gay, Black and having HIV, see www.gayhealth.com.

As we went to press the American Red Cross was planning to issue publications about HIV in African Americans. Check their website at: www.redcross.org

## 3. FOR HELP FINDING HIV ORGANIZATIONS IN YOUR COMMUNITY:

The AIDS Treatment Data Network offers information about national HIV drug assistance programs and other ways to receive free care for HIV. View their website at: www.aidsinfonyc.org.

The AIDS Action website is excellent. You can access it at, www.aidsaction.org.

If you don't have access to a computer, you can call the AIDS counseling hotline: 1-800-590-2437.

Project Inform is dedicating to ending the AIDS epidemic. It sponsors a toll-free hotline for people who have questions about HIV treatments, 1-800-822-7422.

## 4. TO LEARN HOW YOU CAN PREVENT THE SPREAD OF HIV:

The U.S. Centers for Disease Control National Prevention Information Network specializes in prevention. You can call them at: 1-800-458-5231 or log on at: www.cdcpin.org.

Balm in Gilead is an organization that encourages churches to open their doors to people with HIV and to sponsor AIDS ministries. The organization, based in New York City, also provides culturally appropriate, spiritually oriented AIDS prevention and education materials. Call them at: 212-730-7381 or log on: www.balmingilead.org.

## 5. FOR GENERAL INFORMATION ABOUT HIV:

For easy-to-understand information on a wide variety of HIV and AIDS medical and mental health topics, and frank question and answer sessions with HIV physicians, log onto The Body, a commercial website run by the Body Health Resources Corporation, www.thebody.com.

The San Francisco AIDS Foundation offers plenty of information on its website: www.sfaf.org.

Another site for people with HIV that provides a lot of information—about everything from nutrition to opportunistic infections—is www.aids.org. The site also has an extensive bibliography of books about HIV. AIDS.org is dedicated to providing AIDS information on the web.

## 6. FOR INFORMATION ABOUT MEDICATIONS, THEIR SIDE EFFECTS, AND CLINICAL TRIALS:

Contact the National HIV/AIDS Treatment Hotline, 1-800-822-7422 or log onto www.projectinform.org.

How to join a clinical trial:

Contact the AIDS Clinical Trials Information Service, a website sponsored by the National Library of Medicine, at: 1-800-874-2572, or log on at: www.actis.org.

The American Foundation for AIDS Research is a nonprofit, research advocacy organization. The group's website provides information about clinical trials. Log on at: www.amfar.org.

The commercial website, www.centerwatch.com, lists clinical trials that are in need of volunteers.

## 7. FOR SPECIFIC MEDICAL INFORMATION ABOUT HIV, OPPORTUNISTIC INFECTIONS AND AIDS:

The Johns Hopkins University AIDS Service provides up-to-date medical information and question and answer sessions with leading HIV experts. Log on at: www.hopkins-aids.edu.

The federal government sponsors a number of websites about HIV. One is the site of the AIDS Treatment Information Service, of the U.S. Department of Health and Human Services. The site gives a lot of information, but much of it is technical. The website is: www.hivatis.org.

The National Institute of Mental Health, a government research institute in Washington, DC, has information on its website about HIV and brain and central nervous system disease. www.nimh.nih.gov/

The AIDS Information Center at the Veterans Administration also offers clear information about HIV and AIDS. Call them at: 202-273-9206 or log on at: http://vhaaidsinfo.cio.med.va.gov.

## 8. FOR INFORMATION ABOUT APPROVED DRUG THERAPIES:

Log onto the official website of the federal Food and Drug Administration www.fda.gov/oashi/aids/hiv.html. The agency is responsible for approving all prescription drugs, including medications.

If you have encountered a fraudulent HIV treatment, involving drugs, herbal remedies or dietary supplements, you can file an anonymous complaint in your state. To find out how, log onto the Food and Drug Administration's website, which sponsors the program. Also useful in fighting fraud: FDA/State AIDS Health Fraud Task Forces.

## 9. FOR HELP IN DECIDING ON HIV TREATMENT AND STICKING WITH IT:

Log onto the website of The Body, www.thebody.com.

Also try the website of Project Inform: www.projectinform. org. You can call Project Inform's toll-free treatment hotline: 1-800-822-7422.

## 10. FOR INFORMATION ABOUT WOMEN AND HIV:

The federal government's Health Resources and Services Administration sponsors a website about women with HIV. The information is very technical, however, and geared to professional health providers. Log on at: www.hrsa.gov/womencare.htm.

Also try the website: www.blackwomenshealth.com.

Most websites about HIV also have information specific to women and HIV, so try these.

## 11. FOR INFORMATION ABOUT HIV AND GAY BLACKS:

View the website of the Gay Men's Health Crisis, www.gmhc. org. It is one of the largest AIDS advocacy organizations.

Also log onto: www.gayhealth.com.

For information for gay and transgendered people about safe sex and HIV: www.stopaids.org.

## 12. FOR INFORMATION ON TRANSGENDERS AND HIV, SEE:

Transgendered National International: www.tgni.com

FTM International: www.ftm-intl.org

Renaissance Transgender Assoc., Inc.: www.ren.org

## 13. FOR INFORMATION ABOUT HIV/AIDS AND ADDICTION

SAMSHA (Substance Abuse and Mental Health Services Administration of the U.S. Department of Health and Human Services) has a website that leads you to the detox programs you need, at: http://findtreatment.samhsa.gov/

## 14. FOR INFORMATION ABOUT INTERNATIONAL EFFORTS TO FIGHT THE AIDS EPIDEMIC:

The Pangaea Foundation provides excellent information: Pangaea Global AIDS Foundation, 995 Market Street, Suite 280, San Francisco, CA 94103, 415–581–7001 (phone) 415–581–7009 (fax). On line at www.pgaf.org

Harvard University has a website devoted to international AIDS issues. Log on at: www.hsph.harvard.edu/hai

For news about AIDS in Africa, from Africa, log onto: www.allafrica.com/aids.

## 15. FOR INFORMATION ABOUT HOW TO FIND HELP PAYING FOR YOUR HIV TREATMENT AND MEDICA-TIONS:

Log onto the federal government's Health Resources and Services Administration's AIDS website: http://hab.hrsa.gov/getting.html. The agency oversees the major programs that have been set up to help fund HIV treatment, which include the AIDS Drug Assistance Program.

If you don't have access to a computer, you can call the AIDS counseling hotline: 1-800-590-2437.

## 16. FOR INFORMATION ABOUT NUTRITION, FOOD, EATING ISSUES AND FOOD SAFETY:

Turn to the website of the American Dietetic Association, an organization of professional nutritionists who have been certified by their states. The ADA website is: http://hivaidsdpg.org.

Or try: www.aidsnutrition.org, sponsored by the AIDS Nutrition Services Alliance, a group of non-profit organizations that serve people with HIV.

The federal Food and Drug Administration provides information on its website about food safety. Log onto the official website of the federal Food and Drug Administration www.fda.gov/oashi/aids/hiv.html.

Excellent low-fat soul food recipes can be found in:

*The Heart of the Matter: The African American's Guide to Heart Disease, Heart Treatment, and Heart Wellness,* by Hilton M. Hudson, M.D. and Herbert Stern, Ph.D. (Roscoe, IL: Hilton Publishing Company, 2000). The recipes can also be found at: www.hiltonpub.com.

## 17. FOR ADVICE AND INSPIRATION ABOUT FITNESS AND HIV:

Log onto www.HIVfitness.org. The information on the site is provided by an Advanced Certified Personal Fitness Trainer.

## 17. FOR INFORMATION ABOUT ALTERNATIVE MEDICAL THERAPIES FOR PEOPLE WITH HIV:

Be careful! There are many quacks out there who sell dangerous or useless products and only do it in order to get your money. Check with your health provider and local AIDS advocacy organization first before trying anything.

For reasonable information about alternative treatments, log onto a site sponsored by Bastyr University, a college that specializes in alternative medicine: www.bastyr.edu.

## 19. FOR HELP IN FINDING A CONGREGATION NEAR YOU THAT HAS AN AIDS MINISTRY OR WELCOMES MEMBERS WITH HIV:

Contact Balm in Gilead, in New York City. 212-730-7381. www.balmingilead.org.

The AIDS Memorial Quilt is all about remembering and healing. Log onto www.aidsquilt.org.

# INDEX